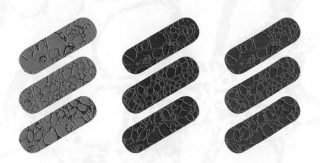

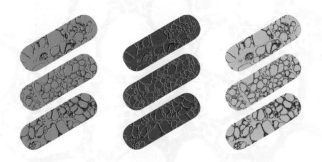

OXFORD BIOLOGY PRIMERS

Discover more in the series at
www.oxfordtextbooks.co.uk/obp

Published in partnership with the Royal Society of Biology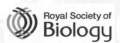

GENETICS IN MEDICINE

≡ OXFORD BIOLOGY PRIMERS

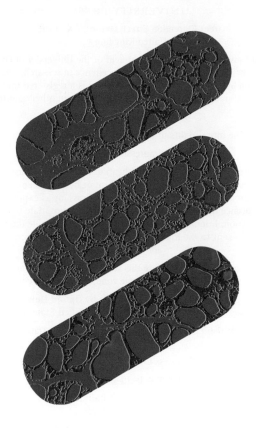

GENETICS IN MEDICINE

Barbara Jennings
Nandu Thalange
Gavin Willis
Subject editor: Aysha Divan

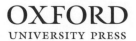

OXFORD
UNIVERSITY PRESS

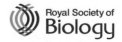

Royal Society of
Biology

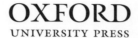

UNIVERSITY PRESS

Great Clarendon Street, Oxford, OX2 6DP,
United Kingdom

Oxford University Press is a department of the University of Oxford.
It furthers the University's objective of excellence in research, scholarship,
and education by publishing worldwide. Oxford is a registered trade mark of
Oxford University Press in the UK and in certain other countries

Published in the United States of America by Oxford University Press
198 Madison Avenue, New York, NY 10016, United States of America

British Library Cataloguing in Publication Data
Data available

Library of Congress Control Number: 2020931792

ISBN 978-0-19-884155-5

Printed in Great Britain by
Bell & Bain Ltd., Glasgow

SERIES PREFACE

Welcome to the Oxford Biology Primers

There has never been a more exciting time to be a biologist. Not only do we understand more about the biological world than ever before, but we're using that understanding in ever-more creative and valuable ways.

Our understanding of the way our genes work is being used to explore new ways to treat disease; our understanding of ecosystems is being used to explore more effective ways to protect the diversity of life on Earth; our understanding of plant science is being used to explore more sustainable ways to feed a growing human population.

The repeated use of the word 'explore' here is no accident. The study of biology is, at heart, an exploration. We have written the Oxford Biology Primers to encourage you to explore biology for yourself—to find out more about what scientists at the cutting edge of the subject are researching, and the biological problems they're trying to solve.

Throughout the series, we use a range of features to help you see topics from different perspectives.

Scientific approach panels help you understand a little more about 'how we know what we know'—that is, the research that has been carried out to reveal our current understanding of the science described in the text, and the methods and approaches scientists have used when carrying out that research.

Case studies explore how a particular concept is relevant to our everyday life, or provide an intimate picture of one aspect of the science described.

The bigger picture panels help you think about some of the issues and challenges associated with the topic under discussion—for example, ethical considerations, or wider impacts on society.

More than anything, however, we hope this series will reveal to you, its readers, that biology is awe-inspiring, both in its variety and its intricacy, and will drive you forward to explore the subject further for yourself.

PREFACE

Our understanding of the genetic basis of disease has grown rapidly over the last decade. The hectic pace of change in genetic science has opened new avenues for the diagnosis and treatment of disease. We have written this book in response to those developments.

The use of genetics in medicine was the ultimate goal of the human genome project, and the resulting technologies have led to the use of whole genome analysis as part of routine healthcare in many countries. Genome analysis has led, in turn, to the potential for individualization of healthcare and we are now on the threshold of the era of personalized medicine.

Genetic medicine is used to diagnose and treat common complex diseases, such as cancer and heart disease that develop over a lifetime; as well as for rare congenital disorders. Because of this, health services urgently need more clinicians and scientists with expertise in genetics.

The complexity of genetics and its terminology and notation are often bewildering. This concise book explains and illustrates genetic medicine using a case-based approach with the help of scientific and clinical scenarios. We wrote the scenarios to trigger the reader's interest and understanding of important research landmarks, key concepts, and medical applications.

There are thousands of examples of both rare congenital disorders and common diseases with an underlying genetic cause. Therefore, this short primer does not serve as a comprehensive textbook describing all of them. Rather, we have written the book to explain core concepts that will help the reader to understand and explore genetic medicine efficiently. There are three ways that the book will be of particular use to undergraduate students.

- The clinical scenarios used in each chapter describe examples of how genetic medicine is already used for the screening, diagnosis, and treatment of disease.

- The research methods used in genetic studies are explained. Understanding study design and terminology will help the reader to navigate the published research literature.

- Databases that systematically document genetic diseases and genetic variants are signposted throughout the book. The linked online resources also have links to freely accessible software. These open resources can support the reader's studies and research through their undergraduate years, and beyond.

Throughout this book, the authors introduce the work and roles of many researchers, physicians, and clinical scientists. We hope that these examples are stimulating, and that they influence the reader's future career plans—perhaps leading to a lifelong interest in genetics and medicine.

The co-authors of this book have worked together for many years teaching undergraduate and postgraduate students at the University of East Anglia (UEA), and conducting research about genetic variation.

ABOUT THE AUTHORS

Dr Barbara A. Jennings BSc, PhD, SFHEA

Barbara Jennings was part of the faculty team that established Norwich Medical School at UEA. She is a senior lecturer and the academic lead for their genetics curriculum. Barbara is a scientist: she completed her PhD about cancer genetics at UEA in 1995, and she has a background in clinical molecular diagnostics for the NHS. Her published research spans cancer genetics, genetic epidemiology, and pharmacogenetics. Barbara is also the course director of a free online course about pharmacogenetics (*Using Personalized Medicine and Pharmacogenetics*).

Dr Nandu K.S. Thalange MBBS, BSc, FRCP, FRCPCH, FHEA

Nandu Thalange graduated from King's College, London in 1988, intent on a career in paediatric endocrinology. During training, Nandu was exposed to a large number of genetic disorders with implications for the endocrinologist which stimulated his interest in this area. For many years he was a senior lecturer at UEA and taught genetics to medical students from the inception of the Norwich Medical School. He remains active as a teacher and clinician and was recently appointed as an honorary Professor of Paediatrics at Mohammed Bin Rashid University, Dubai.

Dr Gavin Willis BSc, PhD, ARCS

Gavin Willis graduated from Imperial College, London in 1985, and began his career in molecular biology and human genetics. He completed his PhD at the John Innes Institute in Norwich, and joined the pathology department at the Norfolk and Norwich University Hospital in 1996, to develop molecular diagnostic markers for leukaemia. Gavin is the principal clinical scientist in the section of molecular genetics, and a specialist in the genetic tests used for the management of families affected by hereditary haemochromatosis.

ACKNOWLEDGEMENTS

The authors want to thank Aysha Divan for her excellent editorial work and for her support and guidance alongside the OUP team.

The authors would also like to acknowledge the following organizations and individuals who have generously contributed to the production of this book.

Many of our illustrations were adapted from original ideas courtesy of Health Education England's excellent Genomics Education Programme. Some images used in Chapters 5 and 6 were courtesy of the Pharmacogenetics Knowledgebase (PharmGKB). Photographs and legends used in Chapters 1 and 6 were provided by Rob Reddick/Wellcome, and Joe Murphy/Norfolk and Norwich University Hospital.

We are grateful to Peter Bickerton, Nana Mensah, and Tom Shakespeare for their time and expertise, and for providing vignettes and interviews that were included in Chapters 1 and 3.

Thank you also, to Robert Plomin for expert advice, and permission to adapt his risk score data in Figure 5.8; to Yoon Loke for his expert advice on pharmacology and illustrations used in Chapter 6; to our peer reviewers for their full and constructive review of our manuscript drafts; and to our undergraduate reviewer, Josh Chambers.

Finally, the authors would like to thank the patients and families who agreed to their cases being discussed anonymously in this text and in teaching sessions.

CONTENTS

1 NUCLEIC ACIDS, GENES, AND GENOMES

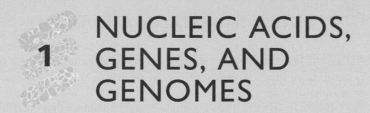

Learning Objectives

By the end of this chapter, you should be able to:

- describe the structure of the DNA molecule and its organization on the chromosomes and in mitochondria of human cells;

- define the human genome and explain the organization of coding and non-coding DNA;

- discuss the role of the HGP and spin-off projects in the advancement of genetic medicine;

- describe and compare the function of RNA molecules in the transcription of genes and their translation into protein sequences;

- describe the regulation of gene expression.

This chapter is an introduction to some of the fundamental concepts that are applied in genetic medicine. The reader will need to understand the structure of DNA, and how the human genome is organized before considering genetic variation and how laboratory tests are used.

Genetic medicine was the ultimate goal for many of the scientists who described the function and structure of DNA, and those who have contributed to the **human genome project (HGP).** These landmarks are discussed here, alongside important new projects and discoveries from the last decade about the regulation of gene expression.

1.1   Deoxyribose Nucleic Acid (DNA)

The main role of deoxyribose nucleic acid (DNA) is the storage and transmission of hereditary information. The information carried in our DNA codes for intermediary and regulatory ribose nucleic acid (RNA) molecules and for proteins.

Its role in heredity is of such fundamental importance that the DNA molecule has an iconic status. Its helical molecular structure is also visually appealing and is symbolized in a range of cultural contexts beyond the classroom, the laboratory, or the scientific text as shown in Figure 1.1.

James Watson and Francis Crick, the scientists who published the succinct description of the DNA molecule in 1953, have become household names and their story is introduced in the Scientific Approach Panel 1.1. Our understanding of the structure of DNA developed incrementally, and the molecular puzzle was solved by interpreting data collected by many geneticists, biologists, and physical chemists.

DNA is a Macromolecule

DNA is a macromolecule that is composed of two polynucleotide strands wrapped around each other to form a double helix. The nucleotide building blocks of DNA are composite molecules; each one consists of a sugar, and a phosphate, and one of four bases: adenine, guanine, thymine, and cytosine. The features of a nucleotide are illustrated in Figure 1.2 (a). The five carbon atoms in each sugar are numbered one prime (1'), 2', 3', 4', 5'. The sugar molecules in DNA and ribose nucleic acid (RNA) are slightly different; DNA has a sugar with a hydrogen group at its 2' carbon atom (deoxyribose), whereas RNA has a sugar with a hydroxyl group at its 2' carbon (ribose).

These nitrogenous bases and their respective nucleotides can be abbreviated to the initials A, G, T, and C. The bases adenine and guanine are purines and the bases thymine and cytosine are pyrimidines. The two strands of a DNA double helix are joined together with hydrogen bonding between complementary bases; adenine bases are always complementary to thymine; and cytosine is complementary to guanine. The purine–pyrimidine pairing rules mean that if we know the sequence of one strand of DNA we can infer the sequence of the complementary DNA strand.

Figure 1.1 Representation of DNA in art and design.

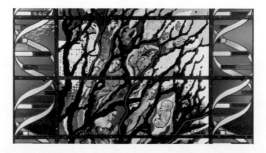

Photograph of a commemorative stained glass window at the Sanger Centre courtesy of Rob Reddick/Wellcome.

Figure 1.2 Nucleotides, polynucleotides, and DNA. (a) A nucleotide consists of a sugar, a phosphate group, and a nitrogen-containing base. (b) The nucleotides in a single strand of DNA are joined by sugar–phosphate (phosphodiester) bonds. Each polynucleotide strand has a polarity that is determined by the orientation of the sugar in its sugar phosphate backbone. (c) In double-stranded DNA the nucleotide sequence of one strand is complementary to the sequence of the other strand.

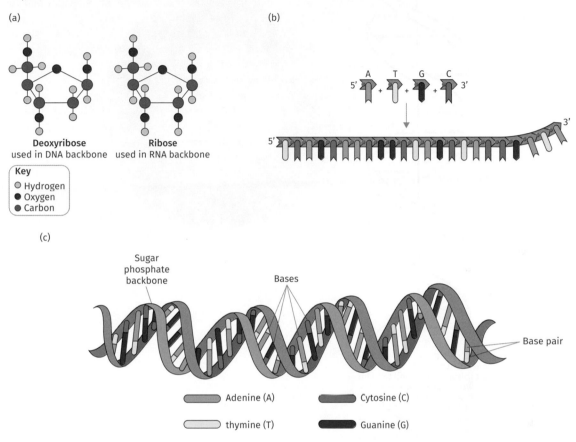

Illustration based on original ideas courtesy of Health Education England's Genomics Education Programme.

Scientific Approach Panel 1.1

A tale of two studies reveals the importance of empirical science and scientific reasoning

Scientific progress and the creation of knowledge depend on the accurate collection of data through experiment and observation (empirical studies) coupled with the use of logic and general principles to draw conclusions and to generate hypotheses (deductive scientific reasoning). The history of how we came to understand the molecular structure of DNA illustrates these aspects of the scientific method rather well.

In April 1953, *Nature* published two letters with iconic illustrations; you can find these back-to-back articles in volume 171 of the journal (see Figure 1.3).

From page 737, James Watson and Francis Crick presented a compelling answer to a longstanding and important question about **heredity**. That is, how does a molecule provide information that can be transmitted

Figure 1.3 Images that defined our understanding of DNA structure in 1953. (a) A hand-drawn figure illustrating a diagram of the DNA molecule from Watson and Crick's letter to *Nature*. (b) A figure illustrating X-ray diffraction data of the B-form of DNA from Franklin and Gosling's letter to *Nature*.

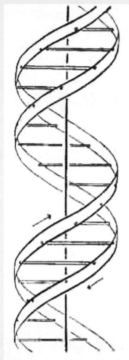
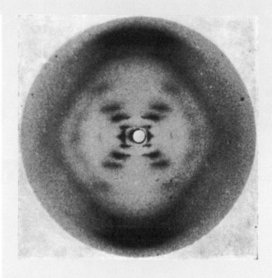

This figure is purely diagrammatic. The two ribbons symbolize the two phosphate—sugar chains, and the horizontal rods the pairs of bases holding the chains together. The vertical line marks the fibre axis

from one generation of cells or organisms to the next generation? The solution was integral to their model for the molecular structure of DNA, which they worked on in the Cavendish Laboratory at the University of Cambridge. Within their paper, they describe the complementary base pairing between specific purines and pyrimidines with the following sentence that is celebrated for its wit.

'It has not escaped our notice that the specific pairing we have postulated immediately suggests a possible copying mechanism for the genetic material.'

From page 740 onwards, of that same volume of *Nature*, Rosalind Franklin and Raymond Gosling described some

of the empirical evidence that Watson and Crick had exploited to understand the DNA structure. Franklin and Gosling's paper presented an image of an **X-ray diffraction** pattern for the **B-form of DNA** that revealed a molecule which was organized as a double helix. Before those results were published, they were shared with the Cambridge scientists by Franklin's colleague at King's College in London, Maurice Wilkins.

The other empirical evidence that Watson and Crick used in their deductive reasoning had accumulated much earlier. For example, the molecule that is known as DNA was discovered and named in the late nineteenth century; and nucleotides were subsequently identified as its building blocks. Furthermore, the complementary base pairing described by Watson and Crick is consistent with a discovery presented by Erwin Chargaff in 1950: which was that there are roughly equal amounts of adenine and thymine in living cells, and roughly equal amounts of cytosine and guanine too.

Once DNA became the prime candidate for providing an organism's hereditary material, a global effort was under way by biologists and chemists who wanted to understand its molecular structure. Data was collected, analysed, and peer-reviewed; and hypotheses were generated and revised. The molecular characterization of DNA was inevitable under these circumstances. Watson and Crick used their understanding of the spatial arrangements of atoms and chemical groups within a molecule (stereochemistry), and scientific reasoning to complete the task. In time, they received a Nobel Prize for chemistry and became household names. Despite the fact that they did not conduct a single experiment with DNA molecules, they had made an incisive and timely discovery. Their 1953 paper is legendary for its clarity and elegance.

Francis Crick recognized the contribution of others, and the privilege and good fortune of being the first to publish their landmark discovery in this quotation from a BBC interview in 1999.

'[Our work on the structure of DNA] was fairly fast, but you know, we were lucky. One must remember, it was based on the X-ray work done here in London started off by [Maurice] Wilkins and carried on by Rosalind Franklin, and we wouldn't have got to the stage of at least having a molecular model, if it hadn't been for their work.'

Task and Discussion Points

- **Read the linked manuscript on the website** (Molecular structure of nucleic acids; a structure for deoxyribose nucleic acid. *Nature* 1953; 171(4356): 737–8) and list four key features of the DNA molecular structure that Watson and Crick proposed.

Semi-Conservative Replication

DNA replication is integral to mitosis and meiosis. Two features of the DNA molecule are illustrated in Figure 1.2 (c), which explain the way this hereditary material can be transmitted accurately from one generation to the next.

- First, the molecule is a double helix made up of polynucleotide strands.
- Second, the nucleotide sequence of one strand is complementary to the sequence of the other strand. This is because a particular purine is always paired with a particular pyrimidine.

Replication produces two daughter DNA strands. This is called semiconservative replication because one of the original polynucleotide strands remains in each daughter molecule along with only one newly synthesized strand. The DNA synthesis phase of cell division and the semiconservative replication of DNA are illustrated in Figures 1.4 and 1.5 (b).

DNA strands separate at multiple sites on each human chromosome and the single DNA strands serve as templates for new daughter DNA strands. The DNA separation occurs, at sites known as **origins of replication** located throughout the genome, during the synthesis (S) phase of the cell cycle in mitotic cells and before meiosis I in the production of germ cells. With every cell cycle, tens of thousands of start sites are established throughout a haploid genome sequence.

The Y-shaped structure in Figure 1.5 (b) is known as a replication fork. Notice the leading DNA strand is synthesized as a continuous fragment; whereas the synthesis from the lagging strand template is synthesized as short stretches, these are called Okazaki fragments. The new daughter strands are constructed

Figure 1.4 Mitosis and meiosis. DNA replication occurs in the synthesis (S) phase of mitosis and meiosis.

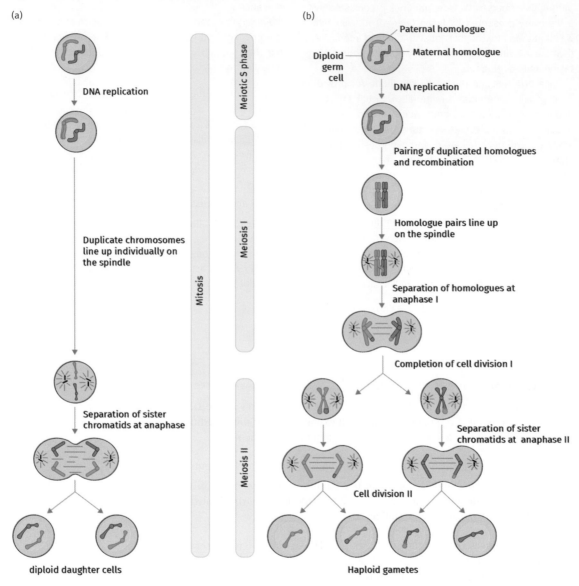

Illustration based on original ideas courtesy of Health Education England's Genomics Education Programme.

by the incorporation of free nucleotides that are complementary to, and can form hydrogen bonds with, the **template strands** (A with T, and G with C).

Enzymes are needed to catalyse the separation and copying of the DNA template strands. These enzymes carry out three distinct roles, which occur in concert rather than as discrete steps:

- **Helicases** and **topoisomerases** allow the transient separation of the DNA strands in the double helix and prevent the tangling of DNA during replication.

Figure 1.5 Semiconservative DNA replication. (a) Diagram of DNA double helix and daughter DNA strands after replication. (b) A diagram of DNA synthesis from an **origin of replication**. One polynucleotide strand is retained (template strand) and nucleotides are added to the newly synthesized leading and lagging strands in a 5′ to 3′ direction. For the lagging strand, short stretches of an RNA polynucleotide prime the synthesis of the daughter strand of DNA by the polymerase enzyme.

(a)

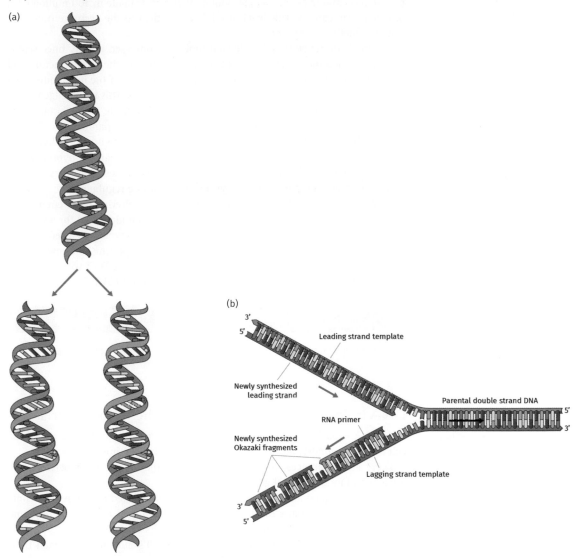

(b)

3′
5′   Leading strand template

Newly synthesized
leading strand   Parental double strand DNA

RNA primer   5′

Newly synthesized
Okazaki fragments   3′

                                    Lagging strand template

3′
5′

Illustration based on original ideas courtesy of Health Education England's Genomics Education Programme.

- DNA polymerases add nucleotides to the growing DNA strand. DNA polymerases can pause if an incorrect base is inserted, so they have an error-correction role.
- DNA ligases join the Okazaki fragments together in the lagging daughter strand.

To facilitate the orchestration and efficiency of synthesis, these enzymes work in multi-enzyme complexes. Once a polymerase binds to DNA, it is very efficient at moving along that strand and adding nucleotides. DNA copying of the human genome has a very high rate of fidelity. Studies of the genomes of parent and child trios reveal approximately one error made in 100 million (10^8) base pair replications. This level of fidelity is critical to the accurate transmission of genetic information.

 See discussions of DNA hybridization, denaturation and synthesis in Chapter 3.

The fields of genetics and molecular biology progressed rapidly once scientists understood the structure of DNA. Understanding its chemical structure and how it is synthesized *in vivo* has led to the development of the techniques used in modern molecular biology and molecular diagnostics. This knowledge has allowed the manipulation and study of DNA molecules in the research and diagnostic laboratories. Double-stranded DNA can easily be separated into the two single polynucleotide strands *in vitro* using denaturation to break the hydrogen bonds. Conversely, complementary single DNA strands can be hybridized to form a double-stranded stretch of DNA and to act as probes or primers for specific sequences. Denaturation and hybridization can be regulated through raising the temperature or lowering it respectively and by altering other conditions. The most efficient and accurate polymerases have been identified for use in the laboratory and together with free nucleotides, these enzymes are used *in vitro* to copy polynucleotide strands. The purine–pyrimidine pairing rules means that if we know the sequence of one strand of DNA (e.g. *AGCTCC*) we can always infer the sequence of the complementary DNA strand (*TCGAGG*).

💡 Key Points

- DNA polymerases have a proof-reading function, so DNA is synthesized with high rates of fidelity at each cell division.

DNA is Found in the Nucleus and in the Mitochondria

> See 1.3 'The Genome' later in this chapter.

Most DNA is packaged with extraordinary compactness into the nucleus of the cell but mitochondria also contain their own relatively minute genome.

There are differences in the organization of the coding DNA between the nuclear and mitochondrial genomes.

The nuclear genome of most human cells (as illustrated in Figure 1.6) comprises twenty-three pairs of chromosomes; each haploid copy of the genome contains approximately 3 billion (3×10^9) base pairs of DNA.

> The mitochondrial genome is also discussed in Chapter 4.

A small amount of DNA is also found in the cell's mitochondria. Each DNA molecule in an individual mitochondrion comprises approximately 17,000 base pairs, organized as a double-stranded circular molecule. It has a linear organization that is more like a bacterial genome than a eukaryotic genome. There are several of these DNA molecules in each mitochondrion, but the exact copy number is variable. The number of mitochondria per cell also varies by cell type.

The chromosomes found in the cell's nucleus are densely packed continuous DNA strands. The DNA is packaged with histone proteins to form chromatin. One method that can be used to analyse the structure and organization of DNA molecules is to study the chromosome complement of the cell with microscopy. The visualization and structure of human chromosomes are discussed in 1.2.

Figure 1.6 An illustration of a mammalian cell and its DNA content. DNA is localized in the nucleus of a cell and in its mitochondria.

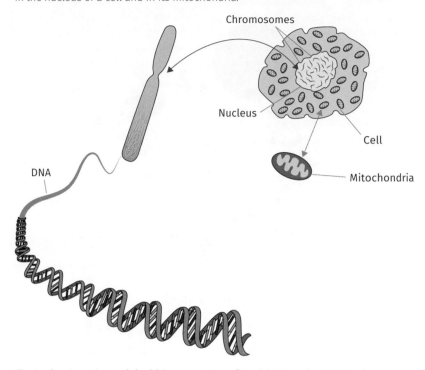

Illustration based on original ideas courtesy of Health Education England's Genomics Education Programme.

1.2   The Karyotype

We have been analysing the human karyotype, which is the number and appearance of the human chromosomes, for nearly a century. The precise cytogenetic techniques that are used have evolved, but some early methods have endured and light microscopy is still used to identify numerical and structural chromosomal abnormalities.

Figure 1.7 (a) illustrates the twenty-four human chromosomes (twenty-two autosomes and the sex chromosomes, X and Y) and the use of the traditional method of analysing the chromosomes from white blood cells. These are grown in the laboratory and treated with a chemical (such as colchicine) to stop cell division when the chromosomes are condensed (i.e. at metaphase or pro-metaphase). Condensed chromosomes can be visualized and analysed by light microscopy if they are spread as a thin layer onto a microscope slide, and stained with a dye (usually Giemsa) to reveal a unique banding pattern for each of them. The word chromosome is derived from the Greek words, *chromos* which means coloured, and *soma*, which means body. Therefore, chromosomes were named because of this ability to take on particular chemical stains. In Figure 1.7 (a) we see the metaphase spread of the human chromosomes from a male. In plate (b), each chromosome from a female karyotype has been cut out

Figure 1.7 Visualization of chromosomes using Giemsa (G) banding and light microscopy.

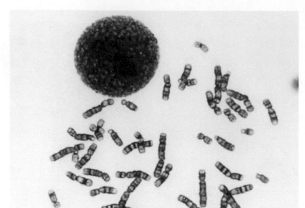

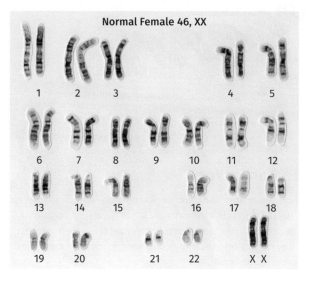

Normal Female 46, XX

and arranged like an idiogram, which is a schematic version of the karyotype. The chromosome pairs are sorted by size and lined up according to the position of the constricted region called the centromere. The **G-banding** patterns can be seen, which is characteristic for each pair of autosomes and each of the sex chromosomes.

The analysis of karyotypes revealed that numerical and structural deviations from this standard chromosome arrangement are often associated with developmental disorders.

Diagnostic genetic labs have gradually reduced their analysis of chromosomes with light microscopy, and employed molecular genetic techniques. This

❯ The application of cytogenetic and molecular genetic techniques are explained in Chapters 3 and 4.

❯ The classification of mutations is described in Chapter 2.

includes the use of fluorescently labelled probes to hybridize with specific chromosome loci and visualization with the use of computerized image analysis systems. In recent years, DNA sequencing has been used to analyse the whole genome systematically for numerical (copy number) and structural variants such as translocations and inversions.

The Autosomes and Sex Chromosomes

The forty-six chromosomes in most human cells are sub-categorized as autosomes (chromosomes 1 to 22) and sex chromosomes (chromosomes X and Y). The sex chromosomes are critical to sex determination, with females having a pair of X chromosomes (XX) and males having an X and a Y chromosome (XY).

The centromere divides the chromosome illustrated in Figure 1.8 into the short (p) arm and the longer (q) arm. The 24 human chromosomes are sub-classified according to the position of the centromere and the relative lengths of the p and q arms.

The chromosomes can be classified with respect to the position of the centromere. The metacentric chromosomes (1, 3, 16, 19, and 20) have a centromere that is roughly in the centre of the chromosomes; the submetacentric chromosomes (2, 4–12, 17, 18, and X) clearly have a shorter p arm; and the **acrocentric** chromosomes (13, 14, 15, 21, 22, and Y) have a centromere that is close to its terminus; most of the DNA in the p arms in these acrocentric chromosomes codes for ribosomal RNA.

The centromere is the constricted region of the chromosome. After DNA has replicated during the **cell cycle** the chromosome can be seen to consist of two identical strands called sister chromatids, which are joined together at the chromosome's centromere.

The cell cycle is illustrated in Figure 1.9, and this term describes a regular pattern of cell division, separated by a period of growth, synthesis, and repair. The longest phase of the cell cycle (interphase) is the period between successive cell divisions. The cell cycle and mitosis are highly regulated in multicellular organisms, which is important for maintaining the integrity of the DNA sequence and the chromosome complement of the cells. Loss of cell cycle regulation is one feature of the cancer cell.

Euchromatin, Heterochromatin, and X-Chromosome Inactivation

The G-banding pattern visible on each chromosome in Figure 1.7 provides some functional information about the conformation of the chromatin and the coding regions of the DNA. The lighter bands are associated with those regions that are actively transcribed.

The basic unit of chromatin is the nucleosome; which is DNA wrapped around a core of eight histone proteins, and short stretches of linker DNA run from one nucleosome to the next. Chromatin exists in two states; as an extended form called euchromatin and in a condensed form called heterochromatin, and respectively, these correspond to the most active and less active regions for transcription. When euchromatin is visualized with an electron microscope, the nucleosomes can appear like beads on a DNA string.

Euchromatin takes up less stain with the G-banding method. The DNA sequences tend to be G/C rich and the chromatin in its extended state, so the DNA is accessible to the cell's transcriptional machinery.

Figure 1.8 Anatomy of a chromosome. The telomeres are the tips of the chromosomes. These terminal repetitive DNA sequences are actively repaired with each cell division to maintain the structure of the chromosome.

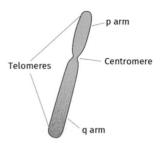

Illustration based on original ideas courtesy of Health Education England's Genomics Education Programme.

❯ Acrocentric chromosomes are revisited in the discussion of Robertsonian Translocations in Chapter 4.

Figure 1.9 The cell cycle. Interphase is the longest portion of the cell cycle, comprising Gap phases (G1 and G2), separated by a DNA synthesis (S) phase. During the mitotic (M) phase, the sister chromatids become visible when the chromosomes are in their most condensed state.

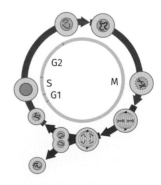

Illustration based on original ideas courtesy of Health Education England's Genomics Education Programme.

❯ See Chapters 2, 5, and 6 for information about cancer and genetic variation.

The darker bands in G-banded chromosomes correspond to regions that have highly packaged heterochromatin, with DNA that is not active in RNA synthesis.

Chemical modifications to histone proteins and the DNA molecule can directly affect chromatin conformation and the transcriptional activity of DNA sequences. These chromatin and DNA modifications are known as **epigenetic** changes. For example, the **acetylation** of particular amino acids in the histone proteins can enhance activity; whereas, the addition of methyl groups (**methylation**) to cytosine residues in DNA can repress transcriptional activity. Epigenetic changes are chemical modifications that alter gene expression without an associated change in the DNA sequence, and can be heritable in **somatic** cells (somatic cells are the cells of the body, rather than the germ cells/gametes).

❯ The importance of epigenetic phenomena and XCI are explored in Chapter 4.

In females, one X chromosome is inactivated at a very early stage of embryogenesis. Once inactivated, the transcription of most genes on that chromosome is also silenced in the successive generations of daughter cells; i.e. **X chromosome inactivation (XCI)** is heritable in the somatic cells. Methylation resulting in XCI balances the dosage of X-linked gene expression between males and females.

 Key Points

- The normal karyotype of most human cells has twenty-two pairs of autosomes and one pair of sex chromosomes.
- A male has one X and one Y chromosome.
- A female has two X chromosomes, but inactivation of one X chromosome in each cell balances the dosage of X-linked genes between the sexes.

1.3   The Genome

The term genome can be defined in several ways. If we describe it simply as *the DNA content of the cell*, this will comprise all of the nuclear DNA, and the 17,000 base pairs of DNA and thirty-seven genes in the mitochondrial DNA.

If we consider the nuclear component only, the genome can be **haploid** for one set of twenty-three chromosomes; or **diploid**, for the full complement of forty-six chromosomes found in most human cells. The haploid human genome contains nearly 20,000 protein-coding genes within its 3 billion base pair DNA sequence.

The Human Genome Project (HGP)

In 1990, the Human Genome Project (HGP) started. The initial aim of the HGP was to sequence an entire human genome, and to define the position of each gene on the 24 chromosomes. Early analysis produced maps and a draft sequence derived from the genomes of selected individuals. Each update since has been a mosaic of sequences derived from the genome analysis of many anonymous donors.

Thanks to the HGP, we have had access to a consensus DNA sequence for almost 100 per cent of our euchromatin since 2003. Over the years, the sequence has become more complete and successive versions are called *assemblies* or *builds*; the latest one is called *Genome Research Consortium human build 38* (GRCh38). These sequences have been used as a reference tool to interrogate the variation that is found between individual human genomes. However, there has been a bias in the selection of participants in genomic studies, so the genomes of people who do not have European or North American ancestry are under-represented. GRCh38 is a much better version for redressing this problem, because it represents alternative versions of some genome regions where there is a lot of diversity between populations.

The HGP was a \$3 billion global effort. It was largely funded by the National Institutes of Health (NIH) in the United States; but also by governments and charities in the UK, France, Japan, China, and Germany. The Medical Research Council and the Wellcome Trust supported the development of the UK's infrastructure for genome analysis, and almost one third of HGP sequencing was completed at the Wellcome Trust Sanger Institute in Cambridgeshire.

Investment in laboratory infrastructure, bioscience careers, and bioinformatics were not the only concerns for the HGP consortium. A portion of the project's overall funding was invested in studies of the ethical, legal, and social implications (*ELSI*) of genome analysis. The over-arching concern was how genetic information might be used to discriminate against people. *ELSI* research explored the protection, privacy, and ownership of genetic data, and the implications of screening for both disease traits and non-disease traits. The possibility that individual gene sequences could be patented for commercial interests was also a concern. One of the HGP principles to circumvent this was to place DNA sequence and gene mapping data into the public domain as rapidly as possible via databases and accessible publications.

❯ which are described in detail in Chapter 3.

Bigger Picture Panel 1.1
Genome projects: from one genome to one million genomes

The HGP led to the development of a new generation of rapid and inexpensive sequencing technologies. The first reference genome took thirteen years and nearly \$3 billion to complete in 2003. Whereas, in 2019, a whole genome sequence can be deciphered in the laboratory and analysed with computer software (bioinformatics) for less than \$1,000 in just a few days.

The impact of the HGP can be gauged from the routine and widespread use of sequencing in medicine today. In many countries, whole genome sequencing is used to identify the cause of rare inherited diseases, and to detect the mutations that drive cancers and affect treatment decisions.

From 2013 onwards, the governments of the fourteen nations tabulated in Table 1.1 and others, had invested billions of dollars in genomic medicine.

In the UK, this included the 100,000 Genomes Project. It was launched by Genomics England (GEL) as a pilot scheme, to create and test health-service infrastructure. The project had a number of parallel aims:

- to identify the underlying causes of a large number of rare diseases suspected to have a genetic origin;
- to test cancer biopsies, and to identify any somatic changes that could be used to sub-classify the disease, and to match the cancer genetics of the patient to any existing treatment protocols;
- to gather research data and any evidence to increase the use of genomic medicine within health services;
- to develop infrastructure, which includes efficient, reliable systems for DNA analysis and increased genetic education for healthcare professionals.

The pilot project was complete in 2018, and because of its success, GEL aims to sequence 5 million genomes from NHS patients over the next five years.

The UK and the other national genomic health projects have all been established to enable the rapid translation of research findings into improved healthcare, and to make the use of medicine more personalized. The success of the HGP depended on rapid data-sharing between

Table 1.1 A list of national projects to develop and advance the use of genomic medicine.

Country	Genomic Medicine Initiative
United States	National Human Genome Research Institute & *All of Us* cohort study
Brazil	Brazil Initiative on Precision Medicine
Australia	Australian Genomics & Genomics Health Futures Mission
Saudi Arabia	Saudi Human Genome Program
Qatar	Qatar Genome
Japan	Japan Genomic Medicine Program
China	China Precision Medicine Initiative
United Kingdom	Genomics England (GEL) 100,000 Genomes Project genomic medicine initiatives in Scotland, Wales, and Northern Ireland
Switzerland	Swiss Personalized Health Network
Netherlands	RADICON-NL rare disease health research infrastructure
France	Genomic Medicine Plan
Estonia	Estonian Genome Project
Finland	National Genome Strategy
Denmark	Genome Denmark
Turkey	Turkish Genome Project

researchers within an international consortium. The translation of genetic science into mainstream medicine will also depend on the exchange of experience and data in this next wave of human genome sequencing: when millions of genomes will be sequenced worldwide.

- **Task and Discussion Point.** Read the participants' stories on the Genomics England webpage (www.genomicsengland.co.uk/about-genomics-england/participant-stories/) and discuss the possible benefits of genome sequencing.

Coding and Non-Coding Elements of the Human Genome

The landscape of the human genome is interesting. It contains fewer protein-coding genes than we once envisaged but many other functionally important elements that can modify phenotypes. Less than 2 per cent of the genome is what we call coding DNA, which is the DNA that comprises the exons of protein-coding genes. However, nearly 20,000 protein-coding genes also contain large tracts of intron sequence and other regulatory DNA sequences. Transcripts from coding sequences can be cut up and re-joined (spliced) in many ways; this is known as alternative splicing. Protein and transcript **isoforms** also occur because of alternative initiation and termination sites for gene expression. This means there are far fewer coding-genes than potential transcripts and protein sequences. This plasticity in the genome is important for tissue-specific gene expression.

In addition to coding DNA, there are thousands of so-called *RNA genes*. These encode RNA molecules that are functionally important but which are not translated into polypeptides. **Non-coding (nc)RNAs**, including those described in Table 1.2, have a variety of roles. Some ncRNAs are critical for fine-tuning gene expression and a few have key roles in embryogenesis or cancer development.

❯ The role of ncRNAs throughout the animal kingdom is discussed in Scientific Approach Panel 1.2.

Some elements of the genome reveal gene evolution; for example, there are many pseudogenes that resemble functional gene sequences but which are not translated into a protein. These could have arisen from gene duplication events and from the silencing of genes that were redundant or surplus to the needs of the organism.

More than half of the genome is taken up with repetitive DNA sequences, and some maintain the structural organization of the chromosomes. The repetitive DNA sequences include those derived from transposons or mobile elements. These are DNA sequences that can, or have, changed position within a genome and they are often duplicated in a sort of 'copy-and-paste' process. Many of the repetitive sequences have lost their ability to move within the genome because of inactivating mutations. Sequences derived from transposons may be a burden to the genome because repetitive sequences can predispose particular loci to higher than average mutation rates because of chromosome misalignment. However, some repetitive sequences may also be under selection pressure because of their role in the advantageous regulation of transcription.

Human genomes are more than 99.9 per cent identical between individuals. The research focus in recent years has been on the wealth of variation, conferred by the sequence differences between our genomes, some of which can be found to be associated with particular traits or phenotypes.

> The classification of genetic variation is discussed in Chapter 2.

One of the aims of an HGP spin-off, called the 1000 Genomes Project, has been to catalogue the functionally important variants with a frequency of > 0.1 per cent in the protein-coding regions of our genomes. This focus is important because most known functional variants, for health-related phenotypes, lie within exons.

Another project that aimed to pick up where the HGP left off is called ENCODE which is the acronym for the Encyclopedia of DNA Elements. ENCODE aims to identify and interpret all of the functional elements of our genome sequence, and its studies show that more than 80 per cent of the genome has some structural or regulatory function in at least one human cell type. GENCODE is a sub-group of the ENCODE initiative, which is annotating and sub-classifying the human (and mouse) gene sequences. Updated GENCODE data is publicly available at their project website (www.gencodegenes.org). The statistics presented in Figure 1.10 are from their version-29 data release and it shows the 2018 sub-classification of 58,721 genes into those that are protein-coding; RNA coding only; and pseudogenes.

Recent genome analysis shows that there are fewer than 20,000 protein-coding genes.

 Key Points

- There are nearly 20,000 protein-coding genes in the human genome.
- The genome also contains pseudogenes, and many functionally important non-coding regions, that are transcribed into long and small non-coding RNA molecules with regulatory and structural functions.

The Protein-Coding Gene

The term gene can be defined as a concept in the study of heredity, and it can also be defined physically within a sequence at a particular locus in a genome.

In 1865, Gregor Mendel published his laws of heredity. He deduced these from his studies of defined phenotypes in generations of garden peas. Mendel concluded that the inheritance of these defined characteristics must be particulate, via pairs of hereditary factors that we now call genes.

Figure 1.10 Gene annotations and classification.

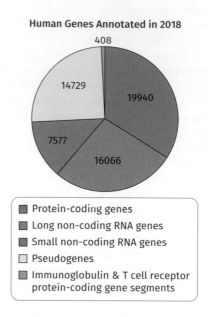

The data presented is derived from: Frankish, A., Diekhans, M., Ferreira, A.-M., Johnson, R., Jungreis, I., et al. (2018). GENCODE reference annotation for the human and mouse genomes. *Nucleic Acids Research, 47* (8 January) (database issue): D766–D773. Published online 2018 Oct 24. doi: 10.1093/nar/gky955

Most human genes are classified as unique single-copy genes that encode polypeptides. The sequence that a protein-coding gene is made of may be as short as a single kilobase of DNA or as long as the *Dystrophin* gene, which is mutated in patients with muscular dystrophy. This gene extends to 2.5 megabases of DNA, and comprises 79 exons with intervening intron sequences. Ninety per cent of gene transcripts can be alternatively spliced, so not all of the exons are translated in the final polypeptide chains. Gene expression is discussed in more detail in 1.4.

❯ 'Gene Expression' later in this chapter.

Exons and introns are two of the physical components of a gene illustrated in Figure 1.11, but there are also upstream (5') and downstream (3') regulatory regions with specific DNA sequence motifs. The first and last exons of a protein-coding gene contain untranslated regions (UTR), called the 5'UTR and the 3'UTR respectively. The ENCODE project has defined regulatory sequences that transcription factors bind to regulate gene transcription. These sequences lie in genome elements described as promoters, silencers, insulators and locus control regions.

💡 Key Points

- Alternative splicing occurs for the transcripts from most coding DNA sequences.
- There are also alternative start and termination sites for gene expression. This means there are far fewer coding-genes than potential transcripts and protein sequences.

Figure 1.11 A diagram of a protein-coding gene. Each gene has exons and introns and regulatory elements. For example near the 5′ end of the coding-DNA sequence, there will be a promoter region with particular sequence motifs, e.g. the TATA box (5′TATAAAAA-3′), to which protein factors bind, to initiate transcription.

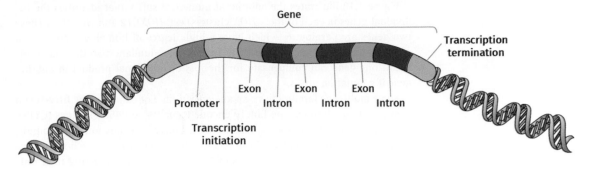

Illustration based on original ideas courtesy of Health Education England's Genomics Education Programme.

Gene Families

Multigene families are made up of groups of genes that have descended from a common ancestor, and that have similar structures and functions. They arise from gene duplication events, which are followed by sequence divergence over time. Therefore, within each family the gene sequences show some degree of sequence homology.

The individual genes of some multigene families lie physically close to each other on the same chromosome, whereas the genes of other multigene families are scattered throughout the genome.

Examples of multigene families include:

- the genes for the immune system proteins, such as the immunoglobulins. This is known as the immunoglobulin **superfamily** because there are many hundreds of genes and gene clusters that encode these proteins;

- the genes of the motor proteins, such as the myosins;

- the genes for some developmental proteins, such as the Homeobox proteins expressed by the *HOX* genes that are illustrated in Figure 1.12.

There are thirty-nine *HOX* genes that encode a class of transcription factors with critical roles in embryogenesis and body patterning. The *HOX* genes are

Figure 1.12 *HOX* genes are found in four clusters. Genes are given universally recognized names by the Human Genome Organization (HUGO) Gene Nomenclature Committee, and each gene in a multigene family is also given a distinguishing suffix. e.g. *HOXA1* is gene 1 in cluster A of the *HOX* genes. This gene is also a paralogue of *HOXB1* and *HOXD1*.

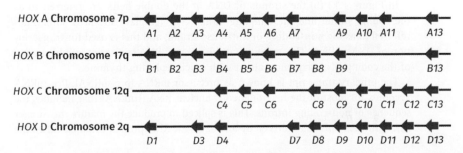

organized as four clusters at different chromosome loci. The genes are named according to the gene clusters A, B, C, and D, which are found at the chromosome loci 7p, 17q, 12q, and 2q respectively.

Figure 1.12 illustrates the additional numerical suffix that identifies the individual genes in each of the 4 *HOX* clusters; e.g. *HOXC12* and *HOXD12*. These two genes are **paralogues** which have a high degree of homology reflecting a common ancestry. This may result in functional redundancy, so that the product of one gene can compensate for the loss of functional product in another gene if a mutation arises.

Some multigene families have an ancient origin. For example, the fifty-seven genes of the *CYP* supergene family encode cytochrome P450 enzymes (CYPs). These metabolize many thousands of endogenous and exogenous compounds, including prescribed medicines and dietary components. There are homologues of the human CYPs in all kingdoms of living organisms, illustrating their universal physiological importance. Such gene sequences, that are found in different species and that are related by descent, are called **orthologues**.

 Key Points

- Data generated by HGP and ENCODE are available via websites and browsers e.g. www.ensembl.org and www.encodeproject.org/

1.4   Gene Expression

Gene expression is the transmission of information from a DNA sequence that results in a gene product. It involves the transcription of DNA sequences into RNA molecules in the nucleus; and, for the protein-coding genes, it results in the **translation** of RNA sequence into polypeptides in the cytoplasm.

> see Figure 1.13 for an illustration.

All diploid cells of an individual have the same genome. However, the gene expression profile varies widely between cells and tissues. Most genes are expressed in a highly regulated fashion; in a particular cell type at a particular time. However, the coding DNA includes **housekeeping genes**, which are expressed in all tissues to provide essential metabolic and physiological cellular functions.

Transcription is the synthesis of a copy of RNA from a gene sequence, which acts as a DNA template.

Like DNA synthesis, transcription requires nucleotide substrates and is catalysed by polymerases; the growing RNA strand is also synthesized in the 5' to 3' direction. Unlike DNA, RNA does not have thymines as one of its pyrimidines, these are substituted by a different nucleotide, **uracil**, during transcription. The initiation of transcription depends on the presence of particular proteins called transcription factors.

In Figure 1.13 (b) the strands of DNA in the double helix are referred to as the coding strand and the template strand. The template strand is sometimes referred to as the non-coding or antisense strand, and this is used for transcription of DNA to RNA. This means that the primary RNA transcript will be a copy of the coding DNA sequence, albeit with uracil replacing thymine.

The primary transcript is known as precursor mRNA (pre-mRNA). Pre-mRNA accounts for most of the heterogeneous nuclear RNA (HnRNA) that includes the sequence of non-coding introns. This is spliced to produce the mature **messenger RNA (mRNA)**. **Splicing** is driven by an enzymatic RNA/protein complex called the

Figure 1.13 (a) A representation of the sites and stages of transcription and translation. mRNA: messenger RNA, tRNA: transfer RNA, amino acids are indicated as purple circles in this diagram. (b) Transcription. The sequence of the template strand is transcribed into the mRNA sequence. The enzyme RNA polymerase converts the DNA sequence into the primary transcript and moves along the template strand in a 3' to 5' direction.

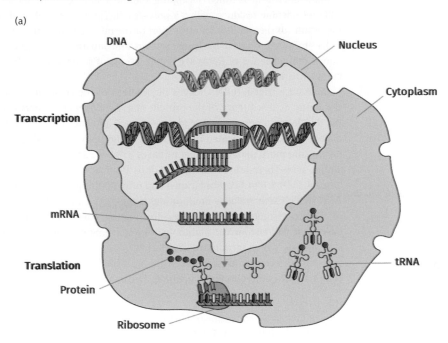

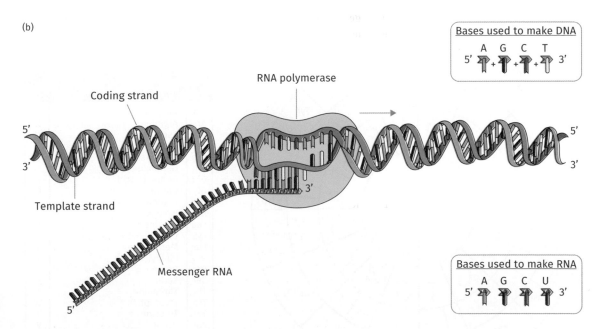

Illustration based on original ideas courtesy of Health Education England's Genomics Education Programme.

spliceosome, which removes the non-coding introns and re-joins the intervening exons at precise sequence boundaries. RNA processing also includes protective modification to the 5' and 3' ends of the molecule. The addition of a modified guanine nucleotide is called 5' capping and the 3' process is the addition of a long chain of adenine residues, called a poly-A tail. These chemical modifications are important for the stability and transport of the mRNA, and its translation.

The mRNA produced by transcription and illustrated in Figure 1.13 (b), is one of many species of RNA; see the functions of some of the other RNA molecules listed in Table 1.2.

Once transcribed, mRNA leaves the nucleus of the cell and is translated into the amino acid sequence of the protein that it encodes. The genetic code defines the relationship between the codon sequence and the resulting amino acid sequence, which is illustrated in Figure 1.14. The DNA code is **degenerate**, which means that more than one triplet of bases (codon) can be translated into a given amino acid. There are 64 possible codons (four nuclcotides read as a triplet of bases = $4 \times 4 \times 4$ (4^3) combinations) and only 20 unique amino acids. The codon AUG (which also encodes methionine) signals the start of the coding sequence of a gene; it therefore determines the reading frame, or particular triplet of bases that will encode the amino acid sequence. Some codons are translated as stop signals, which terminates translation.

A few differences exist between the universal genetic code and the genetic code from the mitochondrial genome. For example, one of the stop signals of

Figure 1.14 The genetic code. (a) This diagram of letter codes illustrates the Universal Genetic Code for the nuclear genome. The first base of a codon is shown in the inner circle; the second base in the next circle, and the permutations of third bases in the third circle. (b) Amino acid nomenclature. Each amino acid name has a three-letter and a single-letter abbreviation.

(a)

(b)

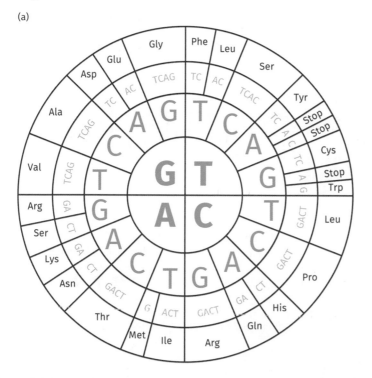

Abbreviations for the amino acids		
Ala	Alanine	A
Arg	Arginine	R
Asn	Asparagine	N
Asp	Aspartic acid	D
Cys	Cysteine	C
Gln	Glutamine	Q
Glu	Glutamic acid	E
Gly	Glycine	G
His	Histidine	H
Ile	Isoleucine	I
Leu	Leucine	L
Lys	Lysine	K
Met	Methionine	M
Phe	Phenylalanine	F
Pro	Proline	P
Ser	Serine	S
Thr	Threonine	T
Trp	Tryptophan	W
Tyr	Tyrosine	Y
Val	Valine	V

the universal code is encoded as the amino acid tryptophan in mitochondrial gene expression.

The site of mRNA translation and protein synthesis is the ribosome, which is a protein and RNA complex found in the cell's cytoplasm.

The Regulation of Gene Expression

Before the HGP was completed, we thought that transcription was mainly confined to coding DNA (i.e. the protein-coding genes) but from large-scale transcriptomic studies, we now know that a much larger proportion of the genome is represented in mature RNA transcripts. Transcriptomics is the study of the complete set of RNA sequences in a particular (sub-cellular, cell, or tissue) sample.

The ENCODE project has analysed the interactions between regulatory molecules and the genome, the sub-cellular localization of RNA species, and the relationship between chromatin structure and gene expression. It has revealed that the regulation of gene expression is dynamic and complex. Studies of the interactions between protein and RNA molecules with the genome have shown the following.

- Multiple transcription factors and RNA molecules co-regulate gene expression in a cell-specific manner.
- Transcription factors (which have DNA-binding domains) regulate gene expression by binding to specific motifs and elements within and around the gene. Some regulatory motifs are a long way from the transcriptional start sites.
- DNA molecules are tightly packaged in chromatin. The regulation of gene expression is also governed by the accessibility of chromatin to the transcriptional machinery. Transcription factor binding to regulatory domains triggers chromatin remodelling.
- Long-range interactions occur between regulatory and coding elements that are separated by many kilobases of DNA on the same chromosome (**cis-regulation**), or that are even on different chromosomes (trans-regulation).

Intra- and inter-chromosomal interactions are facilitated by the spatial organization of the chromosomes, which allow the physical association of the gene sequences and regulatory elements.

We also know that coding transcripts are predominantly localized in the cytosol while many non-coding transcripts are localized in the nucleus. Many regulatory RNAs (see Table 1.2) exert their effect on the gene expression level by degrading mRNA, which is a labile molecule. However, there are other regulatory mechanisms, such as epigenetic modification. The regulation of *HOX* gene expression. Provides one example of this; a long intergenic non-coding RNA called *HOTAIR* is thought to change the DNA methylation pattern in co-operation with protein complexes, and to suppress expression from the *HOXD* gene cluster. Interestingly, the DNA for this transcript lies within the *HOXC* gene cluster on chromosome 12 but silences the *HOXD* gene cluster on chromosome 2; i.e. it is a **trans-regulatory element**.

The small non-coding RNAs called microRNAs (miRNAs) are found in genomes across the animal and plant kingdoms. They are important regulators of gene expression and tissue differentiation.

❯ see Figure 1.12 for a description of this multigene family.

❯ the study of miRNA evolution in mammalian species is discussed in Scientific Approach Panel 1.2.

Table 1.2 Examples of coding and non-coding RNA species that have specific, functionally important roles.

RNA Species	Function
RNA species with a role in protein synthesis:	
• Messenger RNA (mRNA)	• mRNA is a coding RNA. It is the transcript of a coding gene sequence that will be translated into an amino acid sequence.
• Transfer RNA (tRNA)	• tRNA directs the amino acid that it carries into the growing protein chain. tRNA is defined as a non-coding RNA.
• Ribosomal RNA (rRNA)	• rRNA is the RNA content of the ribosome which is the site of protein synthesis. rRNA is also defined as a non-coding RNA.
Small non-coding RNA (snRNA); these include	These RNA molecules do not encode proteins. They regulate levels of protein expression via the degradation of mRNAs or blocking their translation by base pairing with the mRNA. This translational regulation is critical to cell differentiation.
• Short interfering RNA (siRNA)	• siRNAs are double-stranded RNAs of ~ 20–24 base pairs long
• Micro RNA (miRNA)	• miRNAs of ~22 nucleotides are derived from a much larger primary miRNA (pri-miRNA) that form hairpin loop structures.
Long non-coding RNA (lncRNA) e.g. the HOTAIR RNA.	• RNA transcripts > 200 nucleotides long • Regulate gene expression through transcriptional and post-transcriptional mechanisms and epigenetic processes • These long polynucleotides have sequences that lead to secondary and tertiary molecular structures that are linked to their biological functions.

Scientific Approach Panel 1.2
Micro(mi)RNAs, differential gene expression, and evolution

This Scientific Approach Panel is from Dr Peter Bickerton (see photograph) based on research at the Earlham Institute undertaken by Dr Luca Penso-Dolfin in Professor Federica Di Palma's Group.

The human body manages to produce at least 200 different specialized cell types using the same instructions from the same genomic DNA, so there must be some mechanism to differentiate them (see Figure 1.15). In part, that's where miRNAs come in.

Scientists at the Earlham Institute in Norwich are using computer-based methods to compare the sequences of miRNA in different tissue types within and between species. These studies are helping us to understand their role in the evolution of different characteristics in mammals.

We often describe genes being *turned on* or *turned off*. However, the regulation of gene expression can be better understood if it is described as a dimmer rather than a simple on/off switch; the lighting (or expression

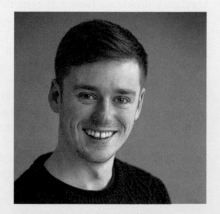

Image courtesy of Peter Bickerton.

Figure 1.15 An illustration of specialized human cells and their relative sizes.

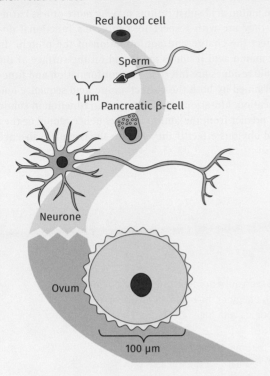

Red blood cell

Sperm

1 μm

Pancreatic β-cell

Neurone

Ovum

100 μm

Illustration based on original ideas courtesy of Health Education England's Genomics Education Programme.

molecule. These mechanisms are not 100 per cent effective, hence the 'dimmer' effect.

Developmentally speaking, miRNAs have an incredibly important role to play. Some miRNAs are themselves more highly expressed in certain cells, so that, in the brain and the heart, for example, the same protein might be expressed, but at different, tissue-specific, levels. For the human genome, there is at least one miRNA for every ten genes, with miRNAs thought to regulate at least one third of human genes.

Research at the Earlham Institute has focused on understanding the role of miRNAs by looking at domesticated animals. The research into five species, namely dogs, pigs, rabbits, horses and cows, shows us where miRNAs could be playing a large role in shaping evolution during domestication; and how they might be responsible for some of the huge changes we see in dogs, for example, in just a short evolutionary timescale. Looking across the five mammal species, using techniques to analyse, annotate and compare sequences, the scientists identified 2088 miRNA sequences, 412 of which were novel. Dogs and cows, in particular, showed a high emergence of species-specific 'seed sequences'. Seed sequences are the bits of miRNA that match exactly the sequence of the mRNA that they target for downregulation. Interestingly, these species-specific seed sequences have target genes that predominantly have a neurological, behavioural or immune related function, which has fascinating repercussions for miRNAs in the domestication process, as all of these processes are positively selected during domestication.

Considering the myriad of shapes and forms of dogs and other domestic animals that we have selectively bred in about 10,000 years, it's clear that there is a relatively quick path towards evolutionary changes. miRNAs may have had an important role in this. The authors conclude that when compared to protein-coding genes, miRNAs represent 'a relatively simple source of innovation'.

in this case) can be finely adjusted. miRNAs have a role between transcription and translation, or sometimes at the stage of translation itself. These tiny molecules, which are approximately twenty-two bases long, just so happen to be complementary to specific mRNA sequences. When a miRNA attaches to the mRNA sequence, the cell may then be instructed to stop protein construction and sometimes even to destroy the mRNA. In animals, what happens is mostly translational repression, while in plants miRNA regulation almost always leads to cleavage of the target

Post-Translational Modification and Protein Function

Translation on the ribosome is not the end of the production-line for newly synthesized proteins. The tertiary structure and function of a protein, its intracellular transport, and its secretion will all depend on post-translational modifications. These may be chemical modifications to particular amino-acid residues or side-chains, such as hydroxylation, carboxylation, and glycosylation. For example, the enzyme activity of the Factor 9 protein, encoded by the

F9 gene, is dependent on the carboxylation (addition of a COOH) group to some amino acids in one domain of the protein.

Mutations that result in amino acid substitutions may be more or less harmful depending on where they are with respect to a protein's functional domains, and how they affect the charge and conformation of the protein. In general, acidic and basic amino acid residues are found on the surface of the protein, whilst hydrophobic residues are internal. The conformation and function of a protein are determined by both the correct amino acid sequence and post-translational modification. Mutations can alter protein function in subtle ways that can be hard to predict from the amino acid sequence alone; or they may have a profound and obvious effect if they lead to the complete absence of an essential protein.

> The functional impact of mutations is explained in more detail in Chapter 2.

Chapter Summary

- DNA replication is described as *semiconservative* because one of the original polynucleotide strands remains in each daughter molecule along with only one newly synthesized strand. DNA is copied with high fidelity from one generation of cells to the next.
- Most of the 3 billion base pairs of DNA that make up a haploid human genome can be found packaged in the chromatin of the nuclear chromosomes. Most human cells have forty-six chromosomes.
- Each mitochondrion in a human cell also has its own genome, with less than 17,000 base pairs of DNA and just thirty-seven genes.
- The human genome has fewer than 20,000 protein-coding genes but many other functionally important regulatory elements, as well as repetitive sequences.
- Epigenetic changes, such as DNA methylation of the X chromosome, can alter gene expression without an associated change in the DNA sequence.
- Gene expression results in a gene product, which can be RNA or protein. Its regulation is complex and dynamic. Alternative initiation and termination sequences as well as alternative splicing mean that there are far fewer coding-genes than potential protein sequences.

Discussion Questions

1.1 Read the manuscript linked to Scientific Approach Panel 1.1, Molecular structure of nucleic acids; a structure for deoxyribose nucleic acid. *Nature* 1953; 171(4356): 737–8 and list four key features of the DNA molecular structure that Watson and Crick proposed.

1.2 Read the participants' stories on the Genomics England webpage: www.genomicsengland.co.uk/about-genomics-england/participant-stories/ and discuss the possible benefits of genome sequencing.

2 MUTATIONS AND GENETIC VARIATION

Learning Objectives

By the end of this chapter, you should be able to:

- describe a range of mutations and how they alter DNA sequences;
- consider the functional impact of mutations on phenotype;
- compare the impact of germline and somatic mutations on health and disease;
- define the key terms used to define genetic variants, including private mutation, rare variant, founder effect mutation, and polymorphism;
- explain how clinical geneticists apply knowledge of human genetic variation in medical practice.

When we observe people, we see phenotypic variation. This includes variation in physical appearance and cognitive skills, as well as variation in disease susceptibility and responses to medicine. Phenotypic variation is often caused by genetic variation, and mutation is the source of the genetic variation between individuals. Every time a cell divides through mitosis, and every time a gamete is produced through meiosis, DNA molecules are copied. This copying can result in errors that are not repaired, which results in mutations that can be passed to daughter cells (**somatic mutations**) or to the next generation of individuals (**germline mutations**).

The Human Genome Project (HGP) was introduced in Chapter 1. The first phase of HGP focused on our similarities and revealed that human genomes are approximately 99.9 per cent identical. As an illustration of our commonality, researchers regularly compare genomes to consensus versions of a **reference genome sequence**, which is one product of the HGP. However, variation between genomes has been the focus of the projects that have emerged from the HGP. Most variants that are common within populations have now been identified, and classified by their impact on the DNA sequence or on gene expression or protein function. In this chapter, we will review some of these genome variants and explain how they can serve as biological markers of disease or treatment response.

2.1   Mutations

A mutation is a heritable change in the nucleotide sequence. Mutations are rare events; approximately one mutation occurs for every 30 million base pairs of human DNA that is replicated. This low mutation rate is because humans, like all eukaryotes, have evolved extensive cellular machinery for accurately copying and proof-reading DNA, and for efficiently repairing DNA damage. However, human cells are exposed to endogenous and exogenous mutagens that increase the rate of DNA damage, and even normal metabolic activity can cause random changes to the DNA structure. Not all DNA damage is subsequently repaired, which makes some mutation inevitable.

The stability of our DNA sequence is partly dependent on DNA repair mechanisms; see the three examples described in Table 2.1. Each of these mechanisms involves enzymatic DNA cleavage, removal of the damaged base/s (excision) and the rejoining (ligation) of the DNA strand breaks.

An individual who has inherited a mutation that affects one of the enzymes with a role in DNA replication or repair may have an increased risk of cancer and other clinical conditions, such as Bloom syndrome and Lynch syndrome. Clinical signs of Bloom syndrome include skin rashes associated with sun exposure and a greatly increased risk of many types of cancer. The underlying genetic cause is an inherited mutation to the *BLM* gene, which encodes an enzyme that is critical to DNA synthesis and repair, called a helicase. Individuals with Lynch syndrome also have an increased risk of several types of cancer, particularly colorectal cancer. Inherited mutations in several genes cause Lynch syndrome; some of the genes are classified as mismatch repair (MMR) genes (e.g. *MLH1*, *MSH2*, *MSH6*, and *PMS2*) because their products are part of the cell's MMR machinery.

❯ MMR is described in Table 2.1.

Most mutations do not occur in coding DNA, and most of those that do are not associated with disease. However, the genetic variation between our genomes results from mutations and we can categorize variants according to the changes we see in the DNA sequence.

DNA Sequence Variation

If we consider the impact of mutations on the base sequence and on chromosomal arrangement and number, there are five types of variation. The effect of each variant on gene expression may be profound if it has an impact on coding DNA (the exome), or regulatory elements within the genome, or if it affects large chromosome regions. However not all coding variants are functionally important, and a new mutation may also have no functional impact if it only alters an **intergenic** region that lacks any regulatory elements.

Table 2.1 Examples of DNA repair mechanisms.

Base Excision Repair (BER)	Nucleases nick the DNA and remove the faulty nucleotide.
Nucleotide Excision Repair (NER)	Nucleases nick the DNA and remove a stretch of DNA that includes the faulty nucleotides.
Mismatch Repair (MMR)	The faulty region can include mismatched bases and small insertions or deletions. This region is excised and repaired.

Tandem Repeats (TRs)

These are short sequences of DNA that are repeated. They are known as mini-satellites (each repeated sequence is 10 to 100 bp long) and microsatellites (each repeated sequence is 2 to 4 bp long). There are typically five to fifty repeats of a sequence, but the number is highly variable between individuals: that is, these loci are highly polymorphic. Most TRs are intergenic and variation has no functional impact on gene expression or phenotype. However, some minisatellites lie in regulatory or coding regions and can have a significant effect on gene function.

Small Insertions and Small Deletions (In/Dels)

These are the insertion or removal of a small number of nucleotides to the chromosome sequence. In coding regions of the genome, these often cause frameshift mutations, when the insertions and deletions are not a multiple of three nucleotides. Figure 2.1 illustrates how these could dramatically alter the amino acid sequence of any expressed protein.

Copy Number Variants (CNVs)

This means gain or loss of very large segments of DNA to and from the genome respectively. It could be the deletion or the duplication of a few thousand bases, or it could result from a change in the number of chromosomes (i.e. *aneuploidy*, such as *trisomy*). These mutations may significantly influence phenotypes by disrupting more than one gene function and more than one biological pathway.

Structural Variants (SVs)

Complex structural variants of chromosomes include insertions, inversions, and translocations and are illustrated in Figure 2.2. If the chromosome breakpoints lie in coding or regulatory regions these mutations can disrupt the whole locus and have a profound impact on the phenotype.

Single Nucleotide Variants (SNVs)

The most common type of genetic variation in human genomes affect single nucleotide pairs and are referred to as point mutation or single nucleotide variant. If the mutation is so common that it is found in 1 per cent or more of the population, it is often referred to as a polymorphism, so an SNV can be a single nucleotide polymorphism (SNP). The recent analysis of large cohorts using whole genome sequencing has revealed that most variants in a human genome are rare variants and private mutations.

Table 2.2 The functional effects of SNV examples on coding DNA. This is illustrated by the mutations highlighted in red to one triplet of bases, and the subsequent impact on the mRNA and protein.

	Reference Sequence	Silent	Nonsense	Missense
DNA codon (coding/ sense strand)	AAG	AAA	TAG	ACG
DNA (template/ anti-sense strand)	TTC	TTT	ATC	TGC
mRNA codon	AAG	AAA	UAG	ACG
Amino acid and protein change	**Lys**	**Lys**	**STOP** (truncated or absent protein)	**Thr**

Figure 2.1 An illustration of the functional impact of frameshift mutations. An insertion of one nucleotide (A) alters the reading frame of the gene and the encoded amino acid sequence is altered. The deletion of one nucleotide (T) alters the reading frame of the gene and the encoded amino acid sequence is altered.

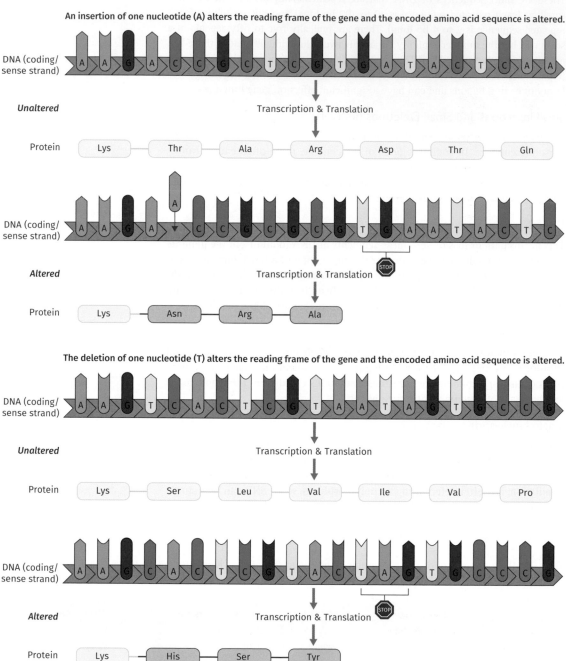

Illustration based on original ideas courtesy of Health Education England's Genomics Education Programme.

Figure 2.2 An illustration of how copy number variants and inversions affect a reference sequence. The loci of the reference sequences labelled A, B, C, and D map to the p arm of this chromosome. The illustrations on the right-hand side of the chromosome illustrate how copy number variants and a structural variant (inversion) can alter the sequence.

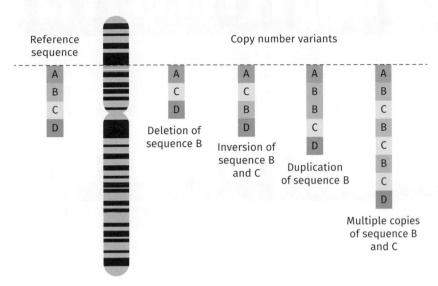

Illustration based on original ideas courtesy of Health Education England's Genomics Education Programme.

The functional impact of the SNV will depend on its location, and whether it affects coding DNA. The impact of a SNV will also depend on the nucleotide change, and how that might affect the encoded amino acid sequence.

To consider how information is transferred from a DNA sequence to its protein product, refer to the fuller description of transcription and translation in 1.4 'Gene Expression'.

The mutations illustrated in Table 2.2 alter the triplet of bases AAG in the coding strand of the reference sequence of a gene. AAG encodes the amino acid lysine (Lys) for example, but some mutations to that particular sequence will be silent, for example, the change in a base from AAG to AAA does not change the resulting amino acid.

Other mutations in the reading frame of an exon may have a profound effect. If changed to TAG, the new sequence will be transcribed as a stop codon as illustrated in Figure 2.3; the mutation will result in the truncation of the mRNA and/ or the amino acid sequence. This type of mutation is called a *nonsense mutation* and its impact is predictably significant. The primary protein sequence may be shorter as a result of a nonsense mutation or it may be expressed at a very low level, or even be absent. This is because there is cellular surveillance for mRNA sequences with premature stop codons, which can cause rapid degradation of the mRNAs.

However, the mutations that we often find hard to predict the significance of are *missense mutations*. These result in a single amino acid change within the encoded polypeptide sequence. For example, while AAG is the DNA codon for lysine (Lys), ACG is the DNA codon for threonine (Thr). This particular change is referred to as a non-conservative change because lysine and threonine have different properties.

❯ To consider how information is transferred from a DNA sequence to its protein product, refer to the fuller description of transcription and translation in 1.4

❯ The degenerate nature of the genetic code is introduced in Chapter 1.

Figure 2.3 An illustration of the functional impact of a nonsense mutation. Nonsense mutations result in the introduction of a stop codon into the nucleic acid sequence.

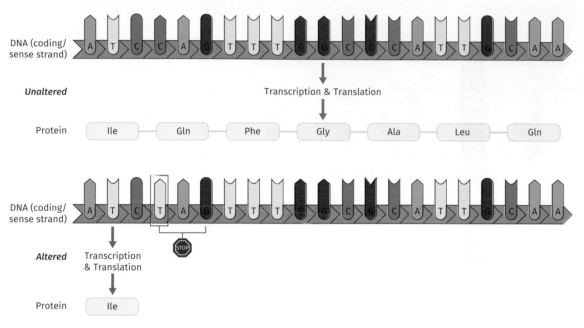

Illustration based on original ideas courtesy of Health Education England's Genomics Education Programme.

> For example; see the common variants of the cytochrome P450 (CYP) family in the discussion of pharmacogenetics in Chapter 6.

Subtle and functionally important variants like these alter the properties of many enzymes and other proteins that affect an individual's disease risk, or their response to prescribed medicines.

The Functional Impact of Mutations

We have considered the categorization of variants by the DNA sequence changes, and their impact on amino acid sequences, in the case of SNVs.

In addition, other terminology, explained in Table 2.3, is used to describe the impact that a mutation has on gene activity, phenotype, or physiology. Some notable examples of mutations that cause rare inherited diseases are listed and described with respect to physiology in 2.7 'Mutations that Cause Rare Disease'.

Genetic Nomenclature

Definitively labelling nearly 20,000 protein-coding genes and describing all mutations that can arise in the 3 billion base pair human genome requires precision. This task is maintained by the human genome nomenclature committee (HGNC), and the Human Genome Variation Society (HGVS). The HGNC and HGVS guidelines are widely followed by clinical genetics services, though shorthand synonyms for particular variants are also used in the research literature and by some laboratories and clinicians.

> See the *HFE* nomenclature in Case Study 5.1 about hereditary haemochromatosis in Chapter 5.

Throughout this book, the official HGNC nomenclature is used to label the human genes, which are presented in upper case, italicized text. Gene names from other species are usually presented in lower case.

Table 2.3 Impact of mutations on the organism.

Mutation	Impact
Lethal Mutation	Causes the developing organism to die prematurely.
	Many congenital chromosomal abnormalities, including most aneuploidies that arise in meiosis, are incompatible with survival **in utero**.
Loss of Function (LOF) Mutation	Reduces or abolishes the activity/amount of the expressed protein.
Null Mutation	This is a type of LOF mutation but the null **allele** results in a complete absence of the gene-product function, and will abolish the physiological activity of the gene.
Gain of Function Mutation	Changes in gene expression pattern. Mutations can increases the activity of the gene; or switch it on constitutively (i.e. permanently, even when physiological conditions are inappropriate) and so it *gains* a new function or expression pattern.
Dominant Negative Mutation	An allele in a heterozygote that blocks or interferes with the activity of the normal copy of the gene. For example, the mutant gene product may disrupt the activity of the normal gene product by dimerizing with it, or it may disrupt the function of a multimeric product.

2.2   *De Novo* Mutations

The term polymorphism is used to describe a mutation that is relatively common in a given population. Conversely, when the term private mutation is used it often means that a new (*de novo*) mutation has occurred in recent history. A private mutation is usually only found in one or a few individuals from a single family. *De novo* mutations are a significant cause of childhood genetic diseases such as neurodevelopmental disorders.

❯ which was introduced in 'DNA Sequence Variation' earlier in this chapter.

The increasing use of DNA sequencing has revealed just how common *de novo* point mutations are. There are between forty and eighty new SNVs reported per individual genome, although only one or two will affect coding regions of the genome. They are usually of paternal origin (i.e. 80 per cent of *de novo* mutations occur during spermatogenesis). Furthermore, increasing paternal age at conception is a risk factor for *de novo* mutations in the offspring. It is thought that the accuracy of DNA repair mechanisms decreases with parental age in general, resulting in more point mutations in particular.

If we consider CNVs, it has been known for many decades that most disease-causing aneuploidies (such as trisomy 21, which causes Down syndrome) also occur *de novo*. Increasing maternal age is a well-established risk factor for the nondisjunction events that lead to aneuploidy in offspring.

For some diseases such as Haemophilia A, a large proportion of the cases are explained by *de novo* mutations of the associated gene. This may be because the DNA sequence has features that put it at high risk of mutations arising, i.e. it is a mutation hotspot. One example of a mutation is an inversion of the X-chromosome which causes many cases of haemophilia A. The underlying flip-tip inversion that causes these mutations of the *F8* gene is explained in Case Study 2.1.

Case Study 2.1
A Common Mutational Mechanism in the *F8* Gene

Haemophilia A is a coagulation disorder that affects ~ 1 in 5,000 male births. The severity of the disease is dependent on the underlying mutation to the large *F8* gene, which is a 186 kb locus that lies on the long arm of the X-chromosome.

We can classify the severity of haemophilia using three phenotypic groups: mild, moderate, and severe. These correlate closely with the level of the Factor VIII protein, which has a critical role in the coagulation cascade. If the protein levels are below 1 per cent of the pooled plasma levels for unaffected people, a severe phenotype results.

Hundreds of different missense, frameshift, and nonsense mutations to *F8* are the causative change in haemophilia families. However, nearly half of cases of severe haemophilia are caused by a particular structural variant called the **flip-tip inversion** that is illustrated in Figure 2.4.

The inversion is caused by a recombination event between a small gene, that lies within the *F8* gene but that is transcribed in the opposite orientation, and a homologous sequence. That mutation is catastrophic because it disrupts the gene sequence and, as a consequence, its expression of the coagulation factor.

It mainly occurs in male germ cells (at male meiosis) and this is probably because in females normal homologous recombination between the two X chromosomes at meiosis prevents this Intrachromosomal recombination event from occurring.

Figure 2.4 Homologous recombination on the X chromosome leads to an inversion that disrupts the *F8* gene. In this diagram, tel = telomere and cen = centromere; arrows indicate the direction of transcription for the gene sequences. The numbers indicate the exons of the *F8* gene. (A) On the long arm of the X chromosome there are three homologous transcribed sequences that are indicated as hatched boxes. One of these sequences lies within the *F8* locus in the intron between exons 22 and 23. (B) The sequence homology between the three homologous sequences leads to intrachromosomal recombination during male meiosis. (C) The result of this is an inversion of the *F8* gene, which disrupts both its structure and expression.

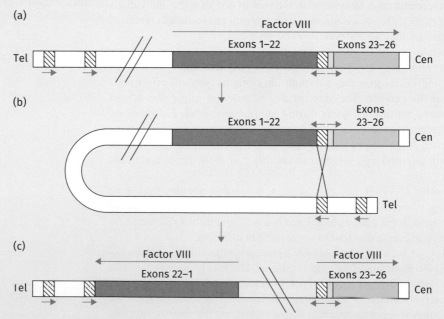

This illustration is based on ideas described by: Purandare, S. M., Patel, P. I. (1997). Recombination hot spots and human disease. *Genome Research*, 7(8), 773–86.

2.3 Mutations, Human Populations, and Haplotypes

Once a mutation occurs, the population frequency, or prevalence, of a genetic variant will partly depend on whether it affects the reproductive success (**fitness**) of an individual carrying that variant. Some mutations may be beneficial but most will be harmful or neutral.

Allele frequencies within populations also depend on human history. As illustrated in Figure 2.5, approximately 100,000 years ago, we know that some modern humans migrated out of East Africa, to other parts of the African continent and to Asia, and from there to the rest of the world. We also know that there have been great population expansions globally since the last ice age, which was nearly 12,000 years ago. Mutations, population mixing, and population bottlenecks (caused by migration, epidemics and other catastrophes) have arisen throughout our history. Some geographical regions were colonized by relatively small migrating groups; in addition, some individuals do not have surviving descendants while others have many. If a population goes through a bottleneck, or was established by just a few individuals, the associated reduction in the genetic variation is called a **founder effect**. Moreover, a mutation carried by one of

Figure 2.5 Global human migrations. The arrows indicate the migration path of modern human populations from approximately 100,000 years ago.

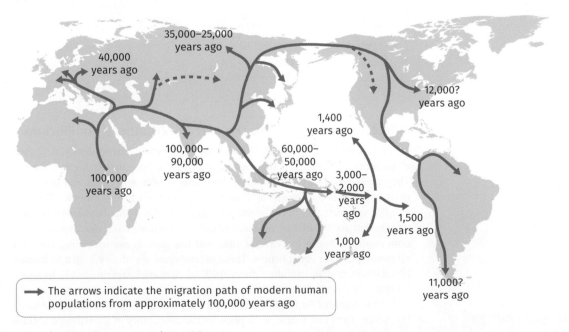

> The arrows indicate the migration path of modern human populations from approximately 100,000 years ago

Figure 2.6 Founder missense mutation p.C282Y (rs1800562) in the *HFE* gene. The variant on the short arm of chromosome 6 was identified in 1996 using a positional cloning strategy.

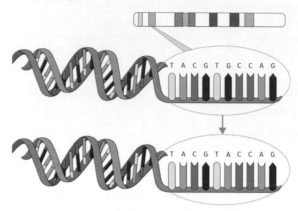

the founders can be passed to future generations and be common in a small isolated population (founder-effect mutation). One example is the p.C282Y variant of the *HFE* gene that is illustrated in Figure 2.6. Most patients with hereditary haemochromatosis are homozygous for this missense variant; it is carried by one in ten Europeans, but is rare in individuals without European ancestry.

As our genes are linked on chromosomes (in the nuclear genome) and in the mitochondrial genome, gene variants are inherited together as blocks of DNA. These blocks of alleles are called haplotypes which are illustrated in Figure 2.7. Tightly linked alleles will be inherited in tandem unless a homologous recombination event (a chromosome crossover event that occurs in meiosis) disrupts the blocks in the nuclear genome. Human history has shaped the resulting haplotype pattern within each genome, and it reflects ancestry or ethnicity.

 Key Points

- Some genetic disorders/mutations are very common in particular populations because all individuals are descended from a small number of ancestors, one of whom had the disorder/carried the mutation.

Alleles, Genotypes, and the Hardy–Weinberg Equilibrium

In 1908, Godfrey Hardy and Wilhelm Weinberg each independently described a mathematical model for the distribution of genotypes in a stable population. They published a formula, defining the numbers of homozygous and heterozygous individuals that would be found in a population in equilibrium. The term equilibrium refers to a freely mixed population; that is a population with no subgroups that are isolated by physical or cultural barriers. HWE also assumes random mating between individuals, that new mutation is not occurring, and that all genotypes have equal fitness. These assumptions are often violated in human populations, and so deviation from HWE is measured experimentally to study mutation and evolutionary forces.

The calculations for HWE are based on the probability of inheriting a particular variant from one parent multiplied by the probability of inheriting a second copy of that variant from the other parent.

	Male Gametes	
	p (A)	q (a)
Female Gametes p (A)	p² (AA)	pq (Aa)
q (a)	pq (Aa)	q² (aa)

If we consider how the alleles are transmitted from one generation to the next for a specific biallelic locus (e.g. for the SNP in the *HFE* gene that is described in Figure 2.6), we can use a Punnett square. The genotypes and alleles of heterozygous parents and their predicted offspring are indicated in the Punnett square that follows:

In this example A = the dominant allele; a = recessive allele.

There are three possible genotypes: homozygous for the recessive allele (aa); heterozygous (Aa); or homozygous for the dominant allele (AA).

In this example, the rare (minor) *HFE* allele also happens to be recessive to the common (major) allele but there are many other examples of a much rarer (minor) allele, which is also the dominant allele.

In the HWE, p and q represent the frequencies of two alternative (major and minor) alleles in the population; their frequencies add up to 100 per cent or 1.

$$p + q = 1, \text{ or } 100\,\%$$

And this relationship between the alleles for a biallelic SNP can be expanded to the following binomial equation:

$$p^2 + 2pq + q^2 = 1$$

Figure 2.7 Haplotypes. The haplotype is a set of linked SNPs on a single chromosome segment; we see an ancestral haplotype and four additional contemporary haplotypes. Most SNPs arise from a single mutation in one individual that is subsequently passed on and spread through the population over generations. The distribution of genetic variants and haplotypes within and between populations, and the frequencies of some reflect ancestral origins.

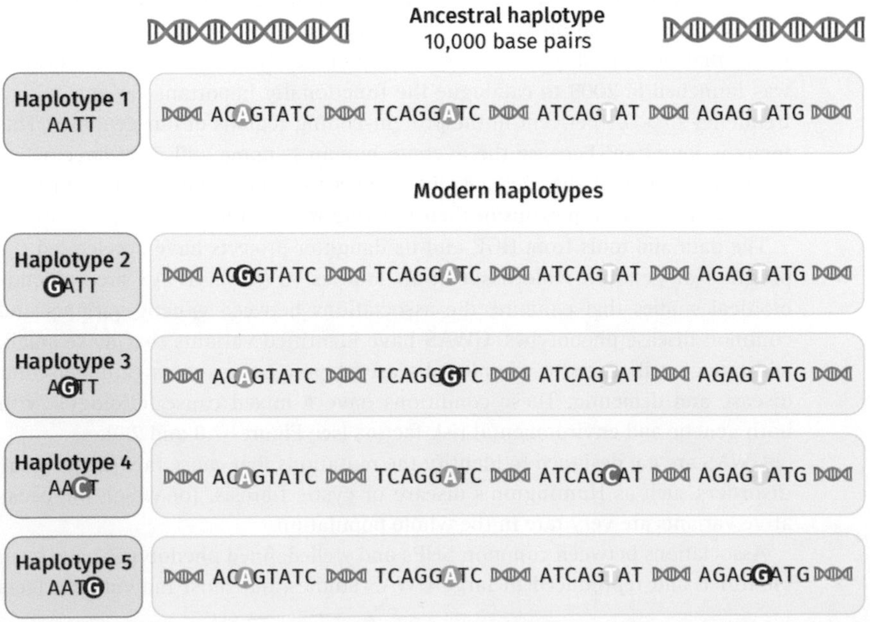

q^2 by convention represents the frequency of homozygous individuals carrying two rarer alleles (aa in the example above); p^2 represents the frequency of homozygous individuals carrying two major alleles (AA).

In a population sample, most of the minor alleles detected will be in heterozyogtes. The frequency of heterozygous carriers (genotype Aa) corresponds to the 2pq term in the Punnett square.

If we know the frequency of a disease-related genotype, the HWE allows us to estimate other genotype and allele frequencies. It is often applied in clinical genetics to predict the population carrier frequency for a recessive monogenic disorder when the incidence of the disease is known. No matter how many generations are considered, the relative frequencies or proportions of the alleles will remain constant in a large, stable population with random mating.

2.4 Databases and Genome-Wide Association Studies

The HGP's reference genome sequence describes approximately 3 billion base pairs of DNA and the position of nearly 20,000 protein-coding genes are mapped to precise loci on each of the twenty-four human chromosomes.

As well as defining the base-by-base genome sequence and the layout of loci on our chromosomes, the HGP has nurtured many spin-off initiatives via the National Human Genome Research Institute (NHGRI). For example, the **HapMap Project** catalogued the common haplotypes. The project described what these variants are, where they occur in our DNA, and how they are distributed among people within populations, and between populations of different ethnicities. The SNPs are also being mapped and are catalogued in their own Single Nucleotide Polymorphism database (**SNPdb**). Within the database, each variant is catalogued against a unique identifier called a refSNP cluster or rs number; for example, the *HFE* SNP described in 2.3 has the identifier rs1800562. A SNP occurs roughly every three hundred nucleotides, which means there are up to 10 million SNPs between the reference sequence and a particular human genome sequence.

This genetic variation was used by researchers to tag sites within the genome that are linked to variations in phenotype. The **1000 Genomes Project** was launched in 2008 to catalogue the functionally important variants with a frequency of > 0.1 per cent in the protein-coding regions of our genomes. This focus is important because the average human genome will only have a few hundred variants of significance with respect to health-related traits and most of those will lie within exons or their flanking regulatory regions.

The data and tools from HGP and its daughter projects have accelerated the progress of **genome-wide association studies** (**GWAS**). GWAS are epidemiological studies that examine the associations between genetic variants and common disease phenotypes. GWAS have identified variants that make small, additive contributions to complex disease phenotypes, such as cardiovascular disease and dementia. These conditions have a mixed cause (**etiology**), with both genetic and environmental risk factors (see Figures 2.8 and 2.9).

GWAS are *not* designed to identify the mutations that cause rare **single-gene disorders** such as Huntington's disease or cystic fibrosis, for which the causative variants are very rare in the whole population.

Associations between common SNPs and well-defined phenotypes have been identified and reproduced in large GWAS studies, but most individual effects

Figure 2.8 An illustration of a genetic association study (GWAS). In GWAS, genome sequences of a large group of people affected by a particular disease are compared with sequences from a second large unaffected group (the control group). If certain variants are found to occur at a different frequency in the disease cases than in the control cases, then they may be associated with the disease risk and/or its cause.

How researchers compare genomic information to identify genetic alterations

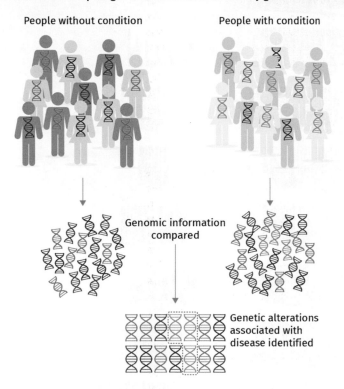

Illustration based on original ideas courtesy of Health Education England's Genomics Education Programme.

of the associated variants are very small; and so have not generated clinically useful biomarkers that can reliably diagnose or predict disease.

However, the usefulness of GWAS has been in the identification of novel associations with genes and molecular pathways that are altered in disease pathophysiology. This knowledge is already opening up possible new targets for drug design and therapeutic interventions.

❯ The application of personalized medicine and pharmacogenetics are discussed in Chapters 5 and 6.

2.5   Genetic Determinants of Disease

In the twentieth century, the application of genetics in medicine mainly focused on rare single-gene (*monogenic)* disorders and chromosome disorders, managed within the specialist clinical genetics departments of large teaching hospitals. Genetic counselling, including the taking and recording of a family history, is a critical aspect of the work of clinical geneticists. The importance of a family history is described in the Bigger Picture Panel 2.1.

Figure 2.9 The impact of the genome-wide association study (GWAS). By January 2019, a curated catalogue of GWAS studies describes nearly 9,000 unique SNP-trait associations. In this diagram, we can see the chromosomal location of individual variants found to be strongly associated with a range of disease markers, from hypertension to drug hyper-sensitivity (**www.ebi.ac.uk/gwas/docs/diagram-downloads**). The genome-wide approach to these studies means that millions of genetic variants are simultaneously analysed by hybridization to microarrays of SNP sequences.

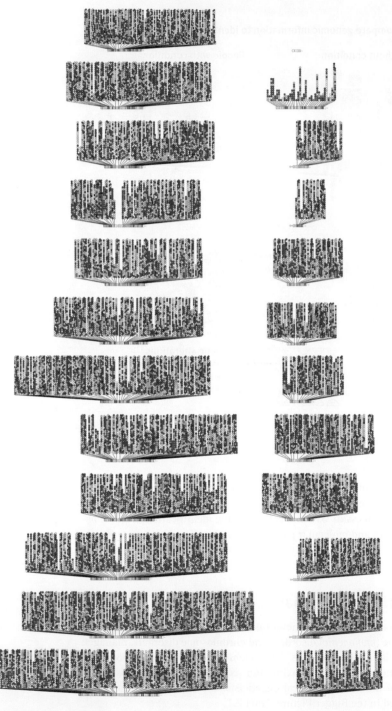

Monogenic diseases arise when a mutation in one gene disrupts the function of that gene, and in general terms, this is the sole or main cause of the disease. Their inheritance patterns are usually predictable and follow Mendelian patterns of inheritance.

This century, genetic medicine will be used much more widely since many common diseases, from cancer to cardiovascular disease and dementia, are now known to have a genetic component. Common, complex traits such as these often result from the cumulative effects of variations in many genes (polygenic), combined with environmental interactions (for example, diet, exercise, exposure to carcinogens). Therefore, while we see family clustering, their patterns of inheritance are not predictable in the way that is observed for monogenic disorders.

The prevalence of monogenic disorders such as Duchenne muscular dystrophy, cystic fibrosis, haemophilia, and Huntington's disease depends on genetic variation in a single gene for each disease. The prevalence of multifactorial disorders such as cancer, cardiovascular disease, and Alzheimer's disease depends on a combination of environmental factors and polygenic genetic variation.

The heritability of a phenotype describes the proportion of the variance observed for a trait that can be explained by genetic factors. There may be additive and interactive effects of many individual genetic variants. It is a population-specific term, which means that heritability can vary over time and between populations.

Another term, genetic architecture, is used to explain the characteristics of all of the individual genetic contributions to a phenotype. Those characteristics include the types and frequency of the variants (alleles) and their impact on the phenotype. Some alleles will have significant functional phenotypic effects (referred to as moderate and major effects in the research literature) and others will have much smaller (referred to as minor) effects. As the understanding of gene regulation has increased, a new model has emerged to explain complex diseases and other traits. In this **omnigenic** model, alleles with very minor effects (referred to as non-zero effects, to illustrate how infinitesimally small they are) from thousands of genes may contribute to the phenotype.

Bigger Picture Panel 2.1
Taking a **family history** —the first genetic test

Taking a family history is a well-established clinical skill. It is often linked to the use of a family tree called the **pedigree diagram**, to accurately record data in a succinct and systematic way. A three or four generation pedigree diagram can reveal patterns of inheritance, and help to predict disease risk for existing and future family members.

The origin of the family history stems from genealogy. From ancient writings, we know that philosophers and authors of sacred texts have been recording family lineages for thousands of years. An interest in family history is deeply ingrained in all human populations.

Recognizing that families shared illnesses, and that the cause went beyond a shared environment, led to an understanding of disease causation. For example, the sex-linked nature of a bleeding disorder that affected males, but that was passed on by mothers, is recorded in the Babylonian Talmud from the second century. It was not until the nineteenth century that a medical doctor described this sex-linked pattern of inheritance for a *hemorrhagic disposition* that we now recognize as haemophilia. Eventually, the cloning of the gene (*F8*) that is mutated in haemophilia A patients depended on the collection of blood samples and detailed histories from large families affected by the disease. The same is true for the identification of genes that cause many **autosomal dominant** and **recessive** diseases.

The practice of taking a genetic family history in a clinical consultation evolved over time, alongside an understanding of the modes of inheritance of monogenic disease. The red flags that should be noted for a role for genetic factors in a patient's disease include:

- an early age of disease onset;
- a multiply affected family (that is there are two or more family members with the same rare disorder);
- multifocal disease (noted in paired organs or in the same organ);
- ethnicity affects the prevalence of the condition.

Medical geneticists and their genetic counsellor colleagues take detailed family histories, and it is a time-consuming procedure. It can take more than thirty minutes to complete a consultation for a three-generation family history, starting from the index case, known as the **proband**.

Drawing up a pedigree diagram creates logistical and ethical problems. For example, the documentation needs to be stored securely in records and may need updating as more information is collected. In addition, if there is a risk of a serious condition affecting other family members, there can be an obligation to contact relatives, who are usually not patients of the consulting physician. There is a universal challenge for genetic medicine, which is that genetic information (derived from history taking or laboratory investigations) has implications for wider family members as well as the patient.

By the early 1990s, professional organizations including a Pedigree Standardization Task Force proposed a detailed system for nomenclature for the Pedigree Diagram. Some of the conventions are illustrated in Figure 2.10; minor stylistic variations for the preferred symbols exist for different clinical genetics organizations worldwide. There have also been updates to accommodate new technologies,

Figure 2.10 Family history (pedigree diagram). Some of the conventions for recording a family history are indicated in this diagram.

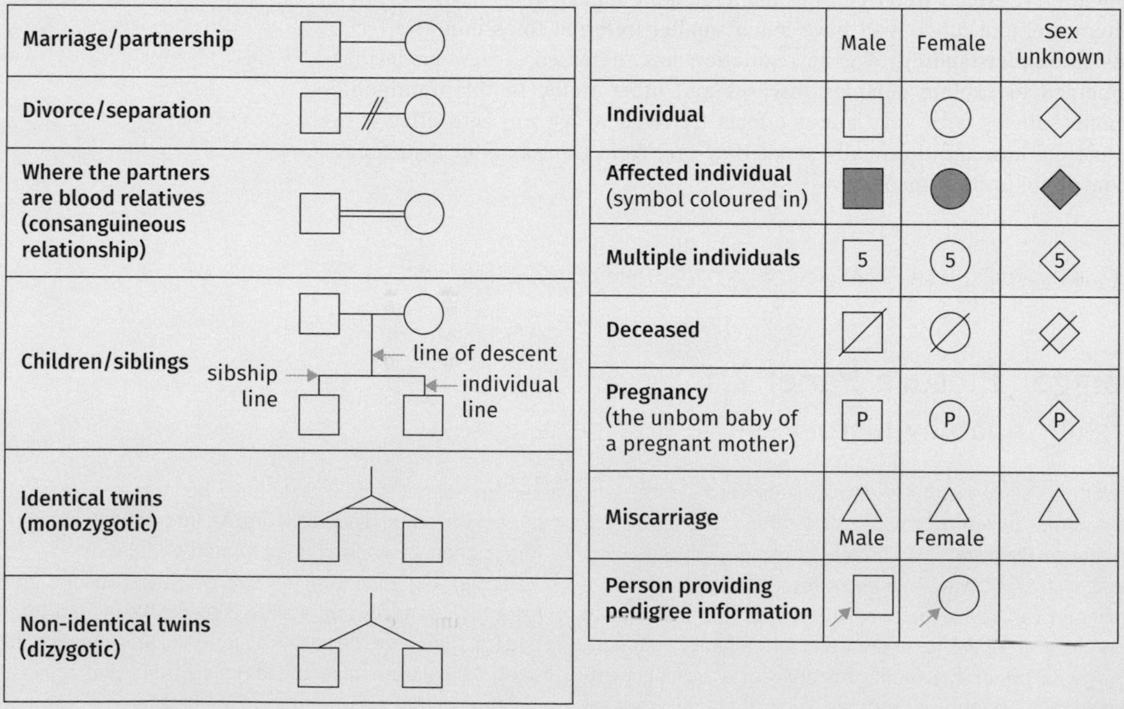

e.g. for recording episodes of assisted reproduction, or pre-symptomatic genetic testing for mutations.

The clinical usefulness (**utility**) for taking a genetic family history includes:

- accurate diagnosis, if the history reveals an underlying genetic cause confirmed with laboratory and clinical investigations;

- identification of family members (of proband) at increased risk of disease;
- risk prediction that can help individuals and couples to make reproductive decisions.

Over the next decade, the clinical practice is likely to adapt further to include data from whole genome analysis and to consider disease with a polygenic cause.

2.6 Somatic Mutations and Cancer

All of the subtypes of mutation described in 2.1 'Mutations' earlier in this chapter can arise in germline cells that go through meiosis or they arise in cells of the body (somatic cells) dividing by mitosis. Somatic mutations that occur and accumulate throughout the life-course underlie the development and progression of some diseases, the most notable example being cancer. Cancer is a genetic disease. Some inherited (germline) mutations are certainly risk factors for the development of some cancers; However, the vast majority of cancers arise because of accumulating **driver mutations** in somatic cells over a lifetime.

❯ see 2.1 for some notable examples.

The mutations that drive the development of cancers affect three classes of genes known as oncogenes, tumour suppressor genes, and DNA repair genes. There are projects that systematically identify and document the mutations that drive the development of many cancer subtypes. These include The Cancer Genome Project and the Catalogue of Somatic Mutations in Cancer (COSMIC) in the UK, and The Cancer Genome Atlas (TCGA) in the US. This work is leading to the identification of new diagnostic, screening, and therapeutic targets cancer genetics is also discussed in Chapters 5 and 6.

❯ cancer genetics is also discussed in Chapters 5 and 6.

Many mutagenic pathways leave an imprint, or mutational signature of SNVs, in/dels, CNVs and SVs in the cancer genome. Large-scale DNA sequencing studies of whole cancer genomes have revealed how a range of endogenous and environmental mutagen exposures lead to particular DNA repair and replication pathways, which in turn result in specific and recognizable types of mutational signature.

💡 Key Points

- Genetic disease can be caused by germline mutations, sporadic chromosome alterations that cause copy number and structural variants, and by somatic mutations.

2.7 Mutations that Cause Rare Disease

Medical genetics can be defined as *the science of human genetic variation applied to health and disease.* Traditionally, clinical geneticists focused on monogenic disorders and congenital malformation syndromes in the translation of that science to rare disorders. The clinical geneticist therefore became the main health-service custodian of knowledge about the mode of inheritance for diseases and the impact of particular genetic variants.

Eighty per cent of rare diseases have an underlying genetic cause. A rare disease is classified as a disorder that affects fewer than 1 in 2,000 of the population. However, if we consider all rare diseases collectively they are common, affecting one in seventeen of the population; therefore, they are often diagnosed and managed by mainstream clinical departments (e.g. cardiology or haematology) as well as by specialist clinical geneticists.

Online Mendelian Inheritance in Man (OMIM) is a curated and regularly updated database of rare genetic disorders. It describes approximately 4,000 individual diseases.

Each OMIM entry is linked to a disease and its associated gene variants. The research that led to the identification of the key genetic variants, many of which will be private mutations, is comprehensively described for each entry.

A few examples of the rare diseases that are managed in both clinical genetics and mainstream settings are described in Table 2.4. The mutational mechanisms and phenotypic effects are listed for each disease.

Table 2.4 Examples of rare genetic disorders.

Disease (Clinical Specialism)	Mode of Inheritance	Gene/Loci	Type(s) of Mutation	Functional Effect of Mutation
Huntington's Disease (Neurology)	Autosomal Dominant	*HTT*	TRs $^\$$	Toxic (harmful) GOF
Duchenne-Muscular Dystrophy (Paediatrics)	X-linked Recessive	*DMD*	In/dels CNVs	LOF
Haemophilia A (Haematology)	X-linked Recessive	*F8*	SV In/del SNVs	LOF
Hereditary Haemochromatosis (type I) (Haematology/ Gastroenterology)	Autosomal Recessive	*HFE*	SNVs *	LOF
Cystic Fibrosis (Paediatrics, Respiratory Medicine)	Autosomal Recessive	*CFTR*	In/dels SNVs	LOF
Myoclonic Epilepsy with ragged red fibres (MERFF) (Paediatrics/ Neurology)	Mitochondrial Disorder	*MT-TK* and other loci	SNVs	LOF
Long QT (LQT) Syndrome (Cardiovascular)	Autosomal Dominant	*KCNQ1* and other loci	SNVs	LOF & Dominant Negative
Ehlers Danlos Syndrome (Rheumatology)	Autosomal Dominant	*COL5A1* and other loci	In/dels SNVs	LOF
Trisomy 22 Syndrome (Fetal Medicine)	*De novo* Congenital Chromosomal	Chromosome 22 loci	CNVs	Lethal *in utero* or soon after birth

GOF: gain of function; LOF: loss of function; SNV: single nucleotide variant; STR: short tandem repeat.

$^\$$ The STRs are CAG (triplet) repeats that result in a polyglutamine tract in the protein.

* Missense Founder mutations of *HFE* are common in northern European populations.

Chapter Summary

- Mutations occur spontaneously and as result of exposure to mutagenic agents.

- Mutations arise during meiosis and so affect the germline. Mutations that occur during mitosis affect somatic cells.

- Because of DNA repair mechanisms, mutations are rare events. Empirical studies show that only one mutation occurs for ~ 30 million base pairs of human DNA that is copied during cell division.

- The functional impact of a mutation will depend on its location, whether it occurs in coding DNA or non-coding DNA, and on how it might affect the gene product.

- Haemophilia A is a coagulation disorder caused by deficiency in factor VIII, which is encoded by the *F8* gene. The most common mutation in severe forms of the disease is the flip-tip inversion.

- A polymorphism is a variant that is relatively common, affecting ≥ one percent of individuals in a population.

- A founder effect arises in a population if all individuals are descended from a small number of ancestors, one of whom carried the mutation/s.

- Whole genome analysis shows that most variants in an individual human genome are rare.

- Harmful genetic variants in a single gene cause monogenic diseases.

- Multifactorial disorders such as cancer and cardiovascular disease are caused by a combination of environmental factors with polygenic genetic variation.

- Genetic counselling is the communication of information and advice about inherited and other genetic conditions. It includes taking a family history and constructing a pedigree diagram.

Further Reading

Timpson, N. J., Greenwood, C. M. T., Soranzo, N., Lawson, D. J., and Richards, J. B. (2018) Genetic architecture: the shape of the genetic contribution to human traits and disease. *Nature Reviews Genetics, 19*(2), 110–24. doi:10.1038/nrg.2017.101

Discussion Question

2.1   This chapter discussed many ways that we can consider a mutation. Read the case study about the flip-tip inversion to the *F8* gene and list the reasons why it might be predicted to result in a severe disease phenotype and why this is a common cause of *de novo F8* mutations.

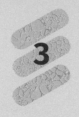

3 LABORATORY TECHNIQUES AND THE SEQUENCING REVOLUTION

Learning Objectives

By the end of this chapter, you should be able to:

- describe how an understanding of DNA structure and synthesis are applied to laboratory methods such as the **polymerase chain reaction** (PCR);

- explain how DNA sequences are analysed to detect pathogenic variants and how **next generation sequencing** (**NGS**) has revolutionized molecular diagnostics;

- compare whole genome sequencing and **whole exome sequencing**;

- explain the terms **non-invasive prenatal testing** (NIPT), **liquid biopsy**, and **variants of unknown significance** (VUS).

Large structural and numerical chromosome abnormalities were traditionally detected using cytogenetics to analyse the karyotype. Over time, emergent molecular genetic methods could detect sub-microscopic variants including single nucleotide variants (SNVs). In recent years, clinicians have started to sequence and analyse many genes simultaneously, and even to interrogate whole genomes in detail. This approach has improved the diagnosis and understanding of many rare diseases and has depended on technological innovation and the use of next generation sequencing (NGS).

NGS has proven itself as a landmark technology because it combines the precision and resolution of molecular diagnostics with the genome-wide perspective of classical cytogenetics; it is also becoming cost-effective. The cost of sequencing has reduced 10,000-fold since the first use of NGS and so the technology has become cheap enough to apply in some healthcare settings.

3.1 Understanding and Exploiting Nucleic Acid Structure

Molecular genetic laboratories have been developed to study the organization of genomes, and the expression and sequences of DNA or RNA. Diagnostic laboratories routinely extract nucleic acids from lymphocytes and other tissues and analyse them using a range of techniques. Molecular genetic tests are applied to many clinical scenarios, including those illustrated in Figure 3.1.

Diagnostic tests are used to help definitively confirm a diagnosis for symptomatic individuals. Screening tests are used to identify individuals with an increased risk of having a particular disease or clinical outcome.

Individual biomarkers, panels of biomarkers, and the analysis of genomes can be used to diagnose and sub-classify disease. Some tests provide predictive information about prognosis, or response to medicines, or disease risk. Others

Figure 3.1 The application of molecular genetic tests in medicine.

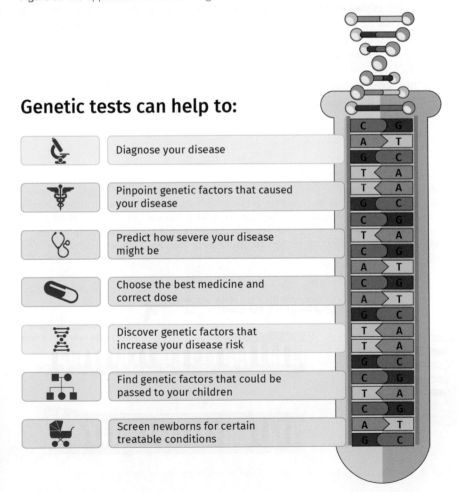

Genetic tests can help to:

Diagnose your disease

Pinpoint genetic factors that caused your disease

Predict how severe your disease might be

Choose the best medicine and correct dose

Discover genetic factors that increase your disease risk

Find genetic factors that could be passed to your children

Screen newborns for certain treatable conditions

Adapted from illustration by National Human Genome Research Institute.

are used for pre-symptomatic and carrier testing for inherited disease or for whole population screening.

Hybridization, Denaturation, and Synthesis

Technical innovation has developed alongside our thorough understanding of the structure and chemistry of the double-stranded DNA molecule and how it is copied and some features are illustrated in Figure 3.2.

❯ The DNA molecule is described in Chapter 1

Many of the key molecular diagnostic methods depend on nucleic acid hybridization steps; that is the formation of double-stranded DNA, or DNA:RNA hybrids from, precisely or partially matched, single strands of DNA or RNA. Using experimental (*in vitro*) conditions that favour stable hybridization between homologous nucleic acid sequences is important for probing for and analysing genetic variants. Exactly matched sequences form the most stable hybrids and so does DNA with a high proportion of GC base pairings (which is often referred to as sequence with a high GC content). Figure 3.3 illustrates that this is because there are three hydrogen bonds between each complementary GC base pair and only two hydrogen bonds between each AT base pair.

The converse of hybridizing or annealing nucleic acids, is their denaturation into single-stranded molecules through the melting of the hydrogen bonds. Temperature, pH and nucleic acid concentration can all be adjusted *in vitro* to favour either denaturation or the specific hybridization of a single-stranded DNA molecule with a complementary nucleic acid (DNA or RNA) sequence. A high temperature; lower salt concentration, and high pH all favour denaturation of the double-stranded molecule.

Figure 3.2 Diagrams of DNA hybridization, denaturation, and synthesis. (a) In the left-hand side of this image is a double-stranded DNA molecule. The single polynucleotide strands have annealed or hybridized. There are hydrogen bonds between the purines and their complementary pyrimidines. The hydrogen bonds have been disrupted or melted in the denatured molecule on the right-hand side of this image. (b) DNA and RNA sequences are copied from template sequences in many molecular genetic assays. In this diagram, we see the synthesis of DNA. Polymerase enzymes are used *in vitro* to catalyse nucleic acid synthesis.

(a)

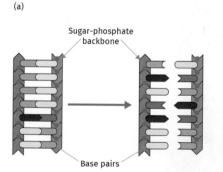

(b)

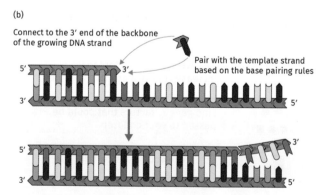

Illustration based on original ideas courtesy of Health Education England's Genomics Education Programme.

Figure 3.3 The number of hydrogen bonds affects the melting temperature of a DNA sequence.

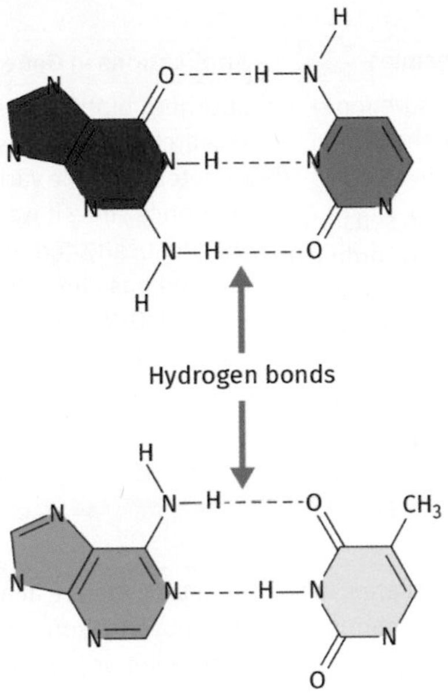

Hydrogen bonds

Molecular Genetic Techniques

The methods described in Table 3.1 and Figure 3.4 have been used to diagnose genetic disease in adults and children, and in fetal medicine The same techniques are also used in microbiology laboratories to diagnose infectious disease, and in oncology departments to sub-classify tumours and monitor response to treatments.

The complementary techniques in the molecular diagnostic toolkit include Southern blotting (to detect the pattern of specific gene sequences that can be precisely cut by particular enzymes called restriction endonucleases); and Northern blotting (to determine the size and amount of messenger RNA transcript in a sample). Both techniques depend on specific nucleic acid sequences hybridizing with each other. The use of microarrays has superseded these techniques for many applications. For example, comparative genomic hybridization (CGH) permits the simultaneous analysis of thousands or millions of target sequences. With microarrays, the molecular geneticist can consider genetic variants across the genome rather than in just a few individual genes.

PCR

Some methods merit particular attention because they have revolutionized research and clinical laboratory practice. The development of PCR was first described in 1986. The use of the technique results in the exponential amplification of short-targeted nucleic acid sequences and it replaced traditional methods of copying DNA fragments by cloning them in host organisms. The sheer efficiency of using PCR as an *in vitro* cloning method led to a commensurate increase in laboratory productivity. PCR has been applied to the diagnosis of genetic disease, the detection of microorganisms, and the ultra-sensitive detection of minimal residual disease during cancer treatment.

❯ PCR protocols and the principles of PCR are described and illustrated in Table 3.1 and Figure 3.4 (c).

Table 3.1 Molecular genetic techniques that include DNA hybridization steps. The protocols and principles of Southern blotting, fluorescence *in situ* hybridization, comparative genomic hybridization, and PCR are compared, alongside their research and diagnostic applications.

Technique	Laboratory Steps and Principles	Applications in Genetic Medicine
Southern blotting	DNA is fragmented using restriction endonucleases that cleave the DNA at specific sequences. Gel electrophoresis is used to separate the negatively charged DNA according to the size of the fragments and the DNA is then denatured and transferred to a nylon membrane. A specific labelled probe for the DNA fragment of interest is then hybridized to the immobilized DNA on the blot. Finally, the pattern of DNA fragments that have hybridized can be visualized.	Southern blotting has been used in research and diagnostic laboratories to detect specific variants in a gene sequence since it was invented in 1975. Diagnostically and in research, this method has largely been replaced by PCR and DNA sequencing methods.
Fluorescence *in situ* hybridization (FISH)	Fluorescently labelled probes are used to hybridize to specific loci on chromosomes. This is visualized using microscopy. The technique is more sensitive than traditional karyotype analysis and can be used on chromosomes prepared at metaphase or interphase.	To detect numerical and structural chromosome abnormalities, including microdeletions and insertions.
Comparative genomic hybridization (CGH)	One fluorescent dye is used to label the DNA being tested, and a different fluorescent dye is used to label a normal or reference sequence. The DNA samples are hybridized and the fluorescent signal is visualized. It is possible to quantify losses and gains of particular loci or chromosome regions. CGH can be carried out on chromosome spreads with specific probes or on microarrays to analyse the genome in more detail.	CGH is used to screen for copy number changes across the genome or to detect specific numerical and structural chromosome abnormalities. Microarray analysis can be used to compare the copy number of genes through analysis of DNA samples, and also to study gene expression in particular tissue samples, through the analysis of RNA samples.
Polymerase Chain Reaction (PCR)	The reaction requires a DNA target template, primers of approximately twenty nucleotides that are complementary to, and anneal to, the flanking sequence of interest, and free nucleotides. Heating and cooling results in cycles of DNA denaturation; primer annealing and extension in the presence of a thermostable polymerase (e.g. Taq polymerase).	PCR is used for the *in vitro* cloning of sequences of interest. Millions of copies of a particular sequence can be produced rapidly and this sequence enrichment is critical for many diagnostic methods used to find mutations.

Figure 3.4 Examples of molecular genetic techniques that include nucleic acid hybridization; fluorescence *in situ* hybridization (FISH) analysis, microarray analysis, and the polymerase chain reaction (PCR). (a) Fluorescently labelled probes are used to hybridize to specific loci on chromosomes. This is visualized using microscopy and can identify copy number variants and structural abnormalities. (b) Microarray analysis is being used in this diagram to compare the RNA profile of one tissue sample from a cancer patient with that of normal tissue. Alterations in the expression profile can provide diagnostic and prognostic information. The microarray consists of oligonucleotide probes arranged in a grid on the solid supports (known as chips). RNA is copied into cDNA using reverse transcriptase. The cancer cDNA is labelled with a fluorescent tag indicated by red and the control (normal) cDNA is labelled with a fluorescent tag indicated by green.

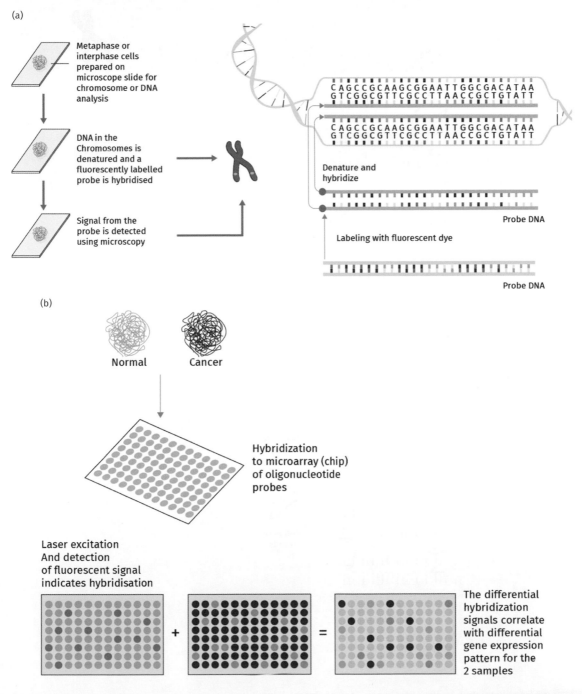

Figure 3.4 (c) The DNA target template, and the primers that anneal to its flanking sequence are illustrated here. PCR is carried out in a thermocycler that can precisely alter the temperature of the reaction vessels. A high temperature denatures the double-stranded molecule, and a lower temperature allows the annealing (hybridization) of the single-stranded primers with the target DNA sequence. A thermostable DNA polymerase rapidly incorporates free nucleotides into new DNA strands. The PCR products are shown in this diagram, after three cycles of denaturation, annealing, and primer extension. The products of one cycle of the PCR become the templates for the next cycle. This results in an exponential amplification of the target DNA sequence.

(c)

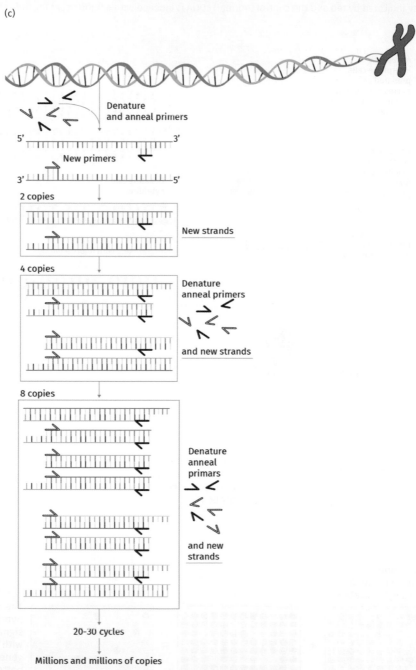

Adapted from illustration by National Human Genome Research Institute.

Interestingly, the theoretical development of PCR only required the lateral thinking of a single scientist and could have occurred years before it happened. This is because an understanding of the individual steps of PCR (DNA denaturation, DNA hybridization, and DNA synthesis) and the necessary *in vitro* reagents had been available for some time. Kary B. Mullis described his necessary leap of imagination to envisage PCR in his Nobel lecture, when he received the 1993 prize for Chemistry.

PCR products are analysed in many different diagnostic protocols. Common, pathogenic SNVs are often distinguished from wild type sequences by using sequence-specific restriction endonucleases. PCR products and/or the products of restriction digestion can then be checked by direct visualization following gel electrophoresis and DNA staining. Automated quantitative PCR systems are used to simultaneously amplify and quantify target sequences. Allele-specific methods can be used to distinguish mutant and wild type products and to identify CNVs. Fluorescent dyes and image analysis are used to detect the products as the PCR reaction progresses in *real time*; hence this method is referred to as real-time PCR. See Figure 3.5 for an analysis of the *HFE* gene using restriction enzyme analysis and allele-specific, real-time PCR.

Key Points

- PCR is widely used in molecular genetic diagnostic laboratories. It results in the synthesis of millions of copies of a DNA segment.
- The reaction requires a DNA template extracted from the tissue of interest; oligonucleotide primers that are complementary to the sequence flanking the region of interest; nucleotides; and a thermostable enzyme.

Over the last decade, the genomics community has embraced another disruptive technology; high-throughput DNA sequencing, which is referred to as next generation sequencing (NGS). As the name suggests, NGS built on other sequencing methods. DNA sequencing methods were first used in the 1970s to determine the nucleotide sequence of particular genes, and they were optimized and linked to bioinformatics to sequence the whole human genome.

3.2   The Principles of DNA Sequencing

In 1975, Fred Sanger described a method for determining the sequence of a DNA strand by copying a complementary strand and monitoring the progress of its synthesis. The method has evolved and been made more efficient with time and technological advancement, but its core principles remain, and are illustrated in Figure 3.6. It is sometimes referred to as enzymatic sequencing, Sanger sequencing or di-deoxy sequencing.

Each version of the technique involves *in vitro* DNA synthesis to copy the template sequence of interest. The reaction mixture includes a short DNA primer to hybridize to the template and nucleotides that are incorporated into the complementary DNA strand by the enzyme DNA polymerase. A proportion of each of the four possible nucleotides, that are included in the sequencing reactions, are modified to allow random termination of DNA synthesis. The modified nucleotides do not have a hydroxyl (OH⁻) group on the 3' carbon, preventing the formation of a phosphodiester bond with another nucleotide. This modification

❯ see Chapter 1 for a description of nucleotide and nucleic acid structure

Figure 3.5 Detection of the *HFE* gene mutation p.C282Y associated with Type 1 hereditary haemochromatosis. (a) Restriction fragment length polymorphism analysis after RsaI digestion, SM; size marker. (b) allelic discrimination and real-time PCR is used to distinguish the wild type homozygous (lanes 1, 4, and 6) heterozygous (lanes 2, 3, and 7), and mutant homozygous (lane 5, indicated by red arrow and circle in a and b respectively) genotypes.

(a)

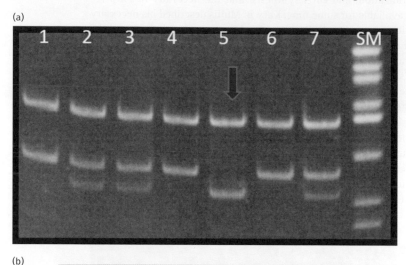

(b)

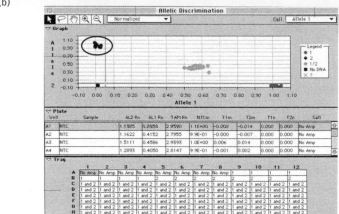

engineers the artificial termination of DNA synthesis at each possible position along a DNA strand. The DNA can be labelled and visualized in a number of ways, including the incorporation of fluorescently labelled nucleotides coupled with the use of high resolution gel-electrophoresis that can fractionate DNA molecules differing in size by only a single nucleotide. Fluorescent signal in the DNA molecules is detected by lasers and the information is processed and can be analysed using computer software.

The automation of the sequencing and bioinformatics steps increased the efficiency of DNA sequencing. This resulted in a rapid fall in the cost per kilobase of DNA sequenced and the use of DNA sequencing became widespread over the years of the Human Genome Project. Instrumentation and analysis software were developed for high throughput sequencing and for smaller-scale applications, including diagnostic testing in hospital laboratories.

The use of DNA sequencing has been critical to the identification of genes that are mutated in rare inherited diseases. The technique is also applied to the routine identification of the variants that cause those diseases in affected individuals

Figure 3.6 The principles of Sanger sequencing. (a) The final DNA sequence can be read by monitoring the fluorescence of each fragment; each of the four modifying nucleotides included in the reaction mixture is labelled with a distinct fluorescent tag; illustrated by the red, green, yellow, and purple asterisks. (b) Sequencing results. The bottom panel shows the identification of a heterozygous missense mutation at base 3050 by Sanger sequencing.

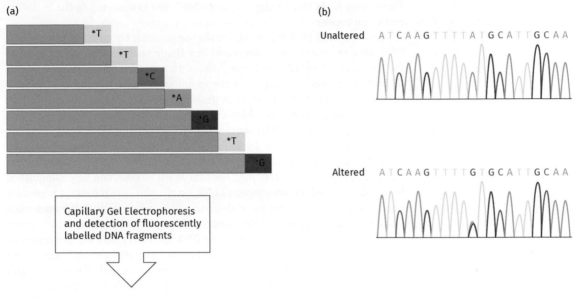

Figure 3.6 (b) based on original ideas courtesy of Health Education England's Genomics Education Programme.

and their families. In diagnostic genetic laboratories, Sanger sequencing is used to analyse gene regions or gene panels to detect particular variants. For now, it is also sometimes used as a gold standard test to confirm variants detected using the newer NGS technology. NGS has made it possible to routinely analyse whole genomes and whole exomes, rather than just individual loci.

3.3 Next Generation Sequencing (NGS)

Rapid and cheap sequencing of whole genomes and exomes is an emergent technology and this coincides it the current revolution in genetic medicine.

NGS technologies employ a range of laboratory instrumentation (such as Illumina's HiSeq) and protocols; there are more than fifty published methods, but they all enable the inexpensive production of very large volumes of DNA sequence data. This is important if the aim is to analyse billions of bases in a whole genome sequence, rather than hundreds or thousands of bases in a particular gene sequence.

Some NGS protocols are based on a sequencing-by-synthesis method that was first described by Shankar Balasubramanian and colleagues in 2008.

NGS steps include DNA template cloning and preparation; sequencing-by-synthesis, through the incorporation of fluorescently labelled nucleotides and imaging to monitor the DNA synthesis; followed by data interpretation and analysis. The analysis requires complex bioinformatics to align and compare the sequence generated with the reference human genome sequence.

Sequencing-by-synthesis usually includes fluorescently labelled nucleotides that reversibly terminate or block DNA synthesis. The imaging step identifies which of the four possible nucleotides has been incorporated, by virtue of its fluorescent dye. The blocking groups on the nucleotides (which result in the termination of the DNA synthesis) are subsequently cleaved, leaving the nucleotides ready for the next sequencing cycle. This widely used method typically results in short sequence reads of 75 to 200 nucleotides. These short reads can be aligned, assembled, and interpreted in the bioinformatics protocols.

NGS is referred to as massively-parallel-sequencing because billions of short DNA sequence reads can be generated in a single analysis. The same region of the genome will be analysed many times and re-sequencing of each stretch of DNA is an important aspect of the technique because it minimizes the risk of misclassifying technical errors as genome variants. This re-sequencing feature of NGS is referred to as a high-coverage, and deep sequencing.

A third generation of DNA sequencing technology has been in use over the last few years; this includes the Oxford Nanopore MinION sequencing, and the method is sometimes referred to as a long-read sequencing. The Nanopore sequencing approach is interesting. The four bases in DNA can be distinguished by measuring conductivity changes as DNA molecules pass through a nanoscale pore; variation in ionic current is detected which corresponds to the nucleotide sequence. The advantages of this method include the ability to complete much longer sequence reads (up to 100 kb of DNA sequence), and the instrumentation used is small, portable and cheap. However, the utility of this sequencing method is currently hampered by a higher overall sequencing error rate, and lower sample throughput than the dominant NGS methods described earlier.

The NGS technology is being used for whole genome sequencing (WGS) and whole exome sequencing (WES), which focuses on the protein-coding elements of the genome only. In Table 3.2 the clinical use of WGS is compared with WES strategies which sequence less than 2 per cent of the genome.

Applied NGS protocols have been developed for RNA sequencing: (RNASeq) by including messenger RNA (mRNA) enrichment and complementary DNA (cDNA) synthesis steps. DNA:Protein interactions are also explored with an adapted NGS

Table 3.2 Comparison of whole genome sequencing (WGS) in laboratory diagnostics with the use of whole exome sequencing (WES).

WGS	WES
The whole 3 billion base pair genome is sequenced and analysed; includes introns and regulatory elements and RNA genes	Only about 30 million bases of the genome is sequenced; the exome comprises the protein-coding DNA
Can detect all variants including CNVs and large structural variants	Useful for the rapid detection of functionally important SNVs and in/dels
Expensive sequencing and data storage	Cheap sequencing and data storage
Can identify pathogenic variants that lie outside the exome	Can identify most (but not all) pathogenic variants found within the exome
Large numbers of variants are filtered in the sequence analysis; each human genome has approximately 5 million variants compared to the reference human genome sequence; a proportion will be rare variants that may or may not have functional and pathogenic importance	Coding variants are filtered in the sequence analysis; each human exome has approximately 30,000 variants compared to the reference human genome sequence; a few hundred of which will be rare variants that may or may not have functional and pathogenic importance

method, to explore epigenetic phenomena; this is called chromatin immunopre-
cipitation sequencing or ChIPSeq. The exquisite sensitivity of NGS also means
that protocols have been developed to analyse single cells and even circulating
fetal DNA and circulating tumour DNA in cancer patients with solid tumours.

❯ see 3.6 'Non-Invasive Testing and Liquid Biopsy'.

 Key Points

- NGS is referred to as massively parallel sequencing because of the vast
  number of DNA molecules that are sequenced simultaneously.
- This has made WES and WGS efficient and cheap and increased its application in medicine.

3.4 Bioinformatics and Variants of Unknown Significance (VUS)

WGS and WES with good sequence coverage, generates roughly 100 gigabytes and
5 gigabytes of data respectively. The raw sequences have to be processed to make
them useful, and storing the raw data is a practical challenge. Bioinformatic analyses are used to detect and annotate variants in the DNA sequence; variants are then
filtered to identify those that are pathogenic with clinical relevance. The variants
of interest may be differences between the nucleotide sequence of the patient and
the human reference sequence (to identify germline variants); or between the DNA
from diseased tissue and normal tissue (to identify somatic or acquired variants).
Applying bioinformatics to clinical genomics is a relatively new field. In Bigger
Picture Panel 3.1, an NHS clinical scientist who is a bioinformatician-in-training
describes the analysis of genomic data.

For diagnostic testing for a single patient or family affected by a genetic
disease, a **bioinformatic pipeline** is created. The pipeline can be defined as a
unique series of computational analyses to translate the nucleotide sequence of
the DNA sample into a clinically actionable result. The steps include:

- the alignment of the DNA sequence with the latest version of the reference human genome sequence;
- comparing the sequences to identify (or call) genuine variants using statistical software and to check the quality of the analysis;
- filtering steps to identify rare variants that are likely to have a pathogenic
  effect;
- filtering steps to identify variants that are associated with the disease
  phenotype within families (for germline mutations);
- filtering and stratification steps to prioritize a review of variants in the
  genes of most interest. This depends on knowledge of disease physiology,
  and from other research or clinical studies of the phenotype.

The biggest hindrance to the usefulness of whole genome sequence data in clinical practice, is that many variants are detected which are inconsequential or
of unknown significance. Incidental and unsolicited secondary findings (that
are not of direct relevance to the primary question) are a common clinical challenge for many diagnostic and screening settings, from radiology to clinical
chemistry; so this is not a problem that is unique to genetics. However, the
big data that is generated by NGS means that the scale of the problem is much

Figure 3.7 A summary of a sequencing and bioinformatics pipeline.

Sample collection

DNA extraction

Library preparation

Enrichment for sequences of interest (e.g. exomes) by hybridisation with labelled probes. The labelled sequence can then be captured by beads for sequencing.

Sequencing

Sequence alignment and variant detection

Variant filtering, clinical interpretation, and reporting

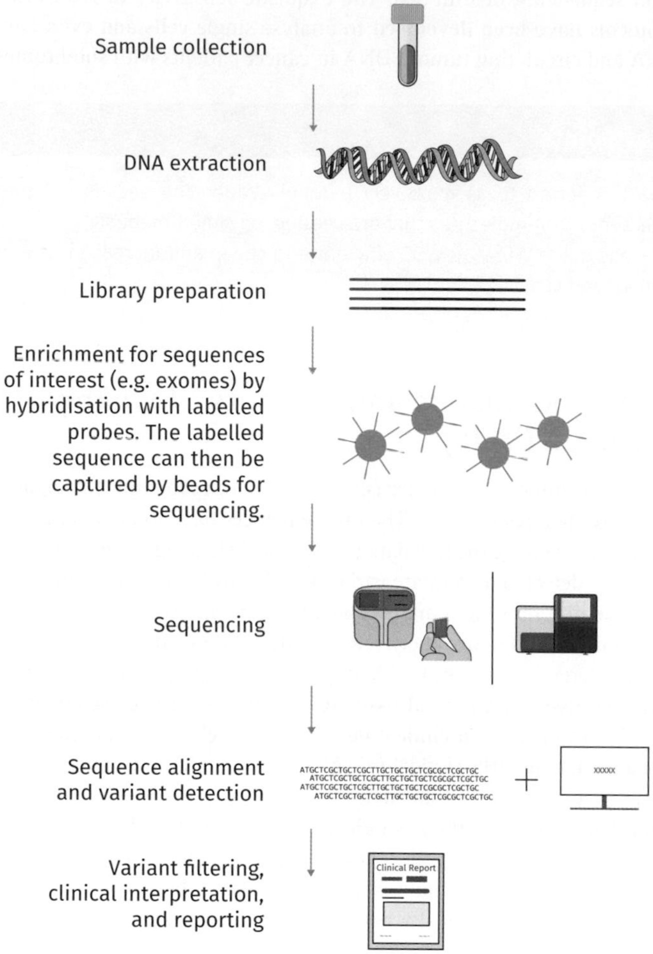

Abhinav Chaudhary/Shutterstock.com.

Bigger Picture Panel 3.1
Nana Mensah (pictured) is a trainee Clinical Scientist at Viapath Genetics Laboratories of Guy's and St Thomas' NHS Foundation Trust.

In this panel, Nana describes the analysis of genomic data from the cell to the computer and clinical report.

Genomic data is the digital representation of an organism's genome. The amount of the genome we capture depends on the sequencing technology we use, but the goal of Clinical Bioinformatics is always to leverage this information for patient care.

The process begins when Clinicians refer patients for genomic testing. First, DNA is isolated from patient samples in the lab, where it is read by high-throughput sequencers. This equipment looks at millions of DNA fragments and produces digital files containing several gigabytes of data per patient.

This data is then processed using bioinformatics 'pipelines'—these are collections of software that

Nana Mensah

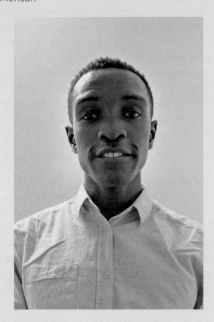

Image courtesy of Viapath Genetics Laboratories; Guy's and St Thomas' NHS Foundation Trust.

transform raw sequence reads into a format ready for human interpretation. This involves quality control steps, such as removing low-quality sequence reads or flagging sample contamination, after which the patient's sequences are mapped to a reference genome. We share 99.9 per cent of our DNA so by identifying where a patient's sequence differs from this reference, we can produce a list of genomic variants, any of which may be the cause of disease.

A list of genomic variants alone is not enough. To know if they are clinically relevant, we have to answer a number of questions: Are there studies implicating this gene with the patient's disease? Does this variant produce a functional protein? How many healthy individuals in the population have we seen with this variant? One of the final steps in a bioinformatics pipeline is to annotate each patient's genomic variants with up-to-date information from a variety of clinical databases.

The role of the Clinical Bioinformatician is therefore highly technical. While we are responsible for developing and maintaining clinical pipelines, there are many services we provide that vary depending on the needs of a given lab. Clinical bioinformaticians can be expected to conduct research into new methods, write software to automate in-house processes, perform one-off analyses and collaborate heavily with other clinical professions.

Communication skills are therefore just as essential as technical skills. As specialists, we make a key knowledge contribution to Genomic Medicine by clearly communicating complex topics to professionals and non-experts alike. For example, our colleagues may need help to understand the cause of an unexpected result, or the nature of any updates to software in the pipeline. With the growing use of machine learning algorithms in bioinformatics, the demand for these communication skills is ever-growing.

greater. NGS inevitably results in a large number of variants of unknown significance (VUS) being found in genes that have been associated with disease risk for rare and common conditions (see Figure 3.7).

3.5 Clinical Diagnostic Applications for NGS

There are two main clinical applications for the sequencing of whole human genomes and exomes. In clinical genetics services, NGS is used to identify causative mutations for rare diseases in symptomatic individuals and their families. In oncology services, NGS is used to sequence genomes from cancer patients to stratify treatment decisions.

Mendelian Genetics/Monogenic Disorders

The use of NGS strategies in research and clinical settings has resulted in a greater understanding of the molecular basis of many rare diseases. This is because underlying mutations were identified for the clinical phenotypes through the use of WGS and WES.

In the clinic, a WES or WGS strategy is often used to identify the cause of a monogenic disease once a putative mode of inheritance has been established. If a new (*de novo*) dominant mutation is thought to be the cause of the disease, trio analysis of the exomes of the affected child and the unaffected parents can be used to identify pathogenic variants that are only present in the child's exome. This has been a very successful strategy for identifying the cause of rare syndromes that result in severe developmental delay. If a recessive disorder is suspected, trio analysis can also be used to identify pathogenic variants carried in a gene by both parents, and for which the affected individual has a homozygous or compound heterozygous genotype.

> for a description of types of mutation see Chapter 2.

Cancer Genomes

NGS is used to identify the somatic mutations that drive carcinogenesis and tumour progression; some of which may be actionable, which means that a treatment exists that is appropriate for the genetic subtype identified. WGS rather than exome sequencing is usually used to identify driver somatic mutations because the mutation types include copy number variants (such as gene amplifications) and structural abnormalities (such as translocations) as well as in/dels and SNVs. Sequencing large numbers of cancer genomes is also improving our understanding of how genetically varied (heterogeneous) cancer subtypes are, and how their evolution allows them to become resistant to conventional treatment protocols.

> as described in Bigger Picture Panel 1.1

The number of whole genomes being sequenced in national public health initiatives is growing rapidly and these efforts span the interface between genetic diagnostic testing and genetic research. In the 100K Genome Project's study of children affected by rare diseases, a definitive genetic diagnosis was identified for some individuals who had previously been investigated inconclusively over many years. This strategy has therefore been welcomed for ending the '*diagnostic odyssey*' for many families affected by rare genetic disease; and so has a project called Deciphering Developmental Disorders. See Case Study 3.1 for a clinical story that has been shared by a family and their consulting physician.

The US Precision Medicine initiative, which involves the sequencing of a cohort of 1 million Americans, also illustrates that health service users are willing to contribute DNA samples and health data for clinical and scientific discovery. Data from these and other initiatives should inform the optimization of diagnostic and screening protocols; and will refine our interpretation of VUS and identification of pathogenic variants. Look at Table 3.3 for a description of how genetic variants are classified.

Case Study 3.1
The diagnostic odyssey—Bethany's story

In this story, Dr Nandu Thalange (a Consultant Paediatric Endocrinologist) reflects on the use of genetic tests, including NGS, in the care of one child with developmental delay and intellectual disability.

Bethany was born by emergency caesarean section at term, after an uncomplicated pregnancy. She had severe vomiting in early infancy and was found to have a relatively large head. Cranial ultrasound showed features of hydrocephalus (excessive accumulation of cerebrospinal fluid), which was treated by insertion of a tube draining excess fluid from the brain into the abdominal cavity.

Subsequently, Bethany was noted to have global developmental delay, hypotonia (low muscle tone), and dystonia (a neurological movement disorder) and she has never gained the ability to walk. Feeding was difficult, and a feeding tube was required to allow appropriate nutrition.

Genetic advice was sought. Her appearance was distinctive, including a prominent forehead (known as frontal bossing), and widely spaced eyes (known as hypertelorism). However, a standard cytogenetic analysis of her karyotype and a subsequent CGH microarray analysis did not identify an underlying cause.

When Bethany was six years old, her mother noticed symptoms of confusion and lethargy in her. These symptoms of chronic low blood sugar (hypoglycaemia) improved with the use of slow-release carbohydrate in Bethany's diet. Following treatment of her hypoglycaemia, Bethany's cognitive function, muscle tone and development markedly improved. Extensive metabolic investigations for hypoglycaemia, including muscle biopsy, showed features consistent with impaired oxidative phosphorylation, but no diagnosis was made.

At the age of eight years, Bethany was entered into the Deciphering Developmental Disorders (DDD) study of whole exome sequencing and ultimately was shown to have a heterozygous mutation in the gene *PPP2R5D*. Several other subjects were identified with *PPP2R5D* mutations and very similar appearance and characteristics.

PPP2R5D is highly expressed in the developing brain and is a key part of a complex system directing the cell cycle. Mutations inhibit its regulatory role, resulting in excessive neuronal proliferation. Subsequently, Bethany was identified as having cerebral folate deficiency and treatment with folinic acid improved her symptoms of dystonia.

The ten years it took for Bethany to receive a diagnosis is very typical of children with intellectual disability syndromes—and even with modern genetic techniques, the majority of patients never receive a diagnosis. Indeed, WES would not have yielded a diagnosis in Bethany's case (without reference to other subjects of the DDD project) because her condition was hitherto undescribed, emphasizing the usefulness of large-scale genetic studies in extending our knowledge of human disease.

Table 3.3 Classification of genetic variants: the classification of variants from pathogenic to benign employs complementary lines of evidence.

Variant	Interpretation
Pathogenic	This sequence change directly contributes to the development of disease. Some pathogenic sequence changes may not be fully penetrant. In the case of recessive or X-linked conditions, a single pathogenic sequence change may not be sufficient to cause disease on its own. Additional evidence is not expected to alter the classification of this sequence change.
Likely pathogenic	This sequence change is highly likely to contribute to the development of disease; however, evidence is not conclusive. Additional evidence is expected to confirm this assertion of pathogenicity.
Uncertain significance	There is insufficient information to support a more definitive classification of this sequence change.
Likely benign	The variant is not expected to have a major effect; however, evidence is currently insufficient to prove this conclusively.
Benign	This variant does not cause disease. Variants that are common in the wider population will probably not be pathological.

3.6   Non-Invasive Testing and Liquid Biopsy

Where medical treatment damages health, it violates a key ethical principle in medicine '*to do no harm*'. However, even diagnostic and screening tests can result in complications, particularly if invasive techniques are used to obtain biological samples for subsequent laboratory tests.

Some prenatal testing strategies can introduce infection and are associated with severe complications; for example, sampling the fetus *in utero* with techniques such as amniocentesis and chorionic villus sampling (CVS) is associated with an increased risk of miscarriage. However, the sensitivity of NGS has provided an opportunity to reduce the volume of invasive prenatal sampling that is used in maternity services. NGS can be used to analyse circulating free fetal DNA (cffDNA) and the DNA can be sampled by simply taking a maternal blood sample. This has resulted in the development of non-invasive prenatal testing (NIPT) protocols to detect trisomies and other genetic abnormalities *in utero* as described in Chapter 4.

Ethical Considerations of NIPT

Prenatal tests to diagnose, or screen for, significant medical conditions and disability can influence the management of a pregnancy in several ways.

First, the results of screening tests may lead to further testing and other interventions during an ongoing pregnancy. Test results may also have implications for managing the delivery of a baby, and/or the early care of the newborn. Finally, the results of tests sometimes lead to decisions being made about whether the parents want to continue with a pregnancy or not.

Each of these, and particularly decisions about the termination of pregnancy, raise ethical challenges.

The ethical principle of autonomy underlies the expectation that tests are only used if consent has been given. For that consent to be fully-informed, healthcare professionals need the knowledge and skills to support women and couples to make informed decisions about the use of prenatal tests.

Ethical principles, such as beneficence (seeking to do good) and non-maleficence (the core principle to *do no harm*), are subjective. Therefore, medical policy and legal frameworks should be discussed and reviewed by the widest possible community. Understanding the lives of individuals affected by the screened-for conditions should be central to any consultation that informs policy and practice. The widespread use of NIPT and NIPD will reduce and may even eradicate some diseases and disability. This possibility raises questions about the way society perceives and cares for children and adults with major disabilities, and about the intrinsic value of human life.

Finally, there is the principle of justice. For healthcare, this means ensuring fair access to health and social care services; that is, for both prenatal services, and for individuals born with significant disability and their families throughout life.

A working group of the Nuffield Council on Bioethics, that considered the use of NIPT in UK healthcare, explored these issues. Please see the Bigger Picture Panel 3.2 for a fuller discussion of their report, which was published in March 2017.

Bigger Picture Panel 3.2

Non-invasive prenatal testing: a conversation about ethical issues and safeguards for the use of genetic knowledge

At first glance, a new technology such as NIPT can be viewed as an entirely positive development. After all, this test just requires a blood sample from the mother, rather than a sample of chorionic villus or amniocytes; and so the sampling is intrinsically safer for both mother and fetus.

However, before a range of NIPT and NIPD services were introduced within the NHS, there were complexities to consider including the ethical principles discussed in 'Ethical Considerations of NIPT'. Therefore, a report was commissioned from a working group of the Nuffield Council on Bioethics. Their remit was to consult widely and to consider the ethical, legal, and regulatory implications of recent (and predicted future) developments with the use of NIPT in healthcare.

The findings were published in March 2017, and disseminated. The report (*Non-invasive prenatal testing: ethical issues*) can be found on the organization's website: www.nuffieldbioethics.org

In their executive summary, the working group made a series of observations and recommendations for policy development, including the following.

- They noted the advantages of NIPT over current screening and diagnostic methods, particularly with respect to reducing miscarriage rates and providing users with earlier results. They also noted the range of serious conditions and impairments that NIPT and NIPD could be used to test for, from trisomies, to sex-linked and monogenic disorders.
- They recommended that women and couples should have access to NIPT to screen for or diagnose those significant medical conditions and impairments that manifest at birth or in childhood. But the group did not recommend its use for less significant or adult onset conditions and they cautioned against missiion creep, and in particular highlighted its potential use for sex discrimination.
- To ensure fully informed consent, the group recommended that high-quality education and training must be compulsory for all professionals involved in NHS screening.

Professor Tom Shakespeare

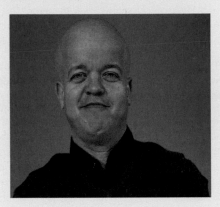

Image courtesy of Tom Shakespeare.

- Ethical values were explored by using surveys, meetings, and interviews with stakeholders including service users. One of the issues emphasized, is that if NIPT leads to a reduction in the number of people born with and living with disability, it could lead to limited resources being invested in research and care for people with genetic conditions.

The working group was chaired by Tom Shakespeare, who is the Professor of Disability Research at the London School of Hygiene and Tropical Medicine.

In autumn, 2018, the author asked Tom to reflect on the likely impact of NIPT in both publicly funded and private health services. This is a narrative summary of Tom's response.

Considering the advantages of NIPT

'Cell-free fetal DNA (cffDNA) tests appear to be quick, easy and are reliable tests.

They avoid the risk of iatrogenic miscarriage (i.e. miscarriage caused by the invasive sampling procedure).

They can be extended to other conditions and situations—such as sex selection. They appear to be an improvement on serum testing. So, they have a role in promoting informed consent.'

What are the potential disadvantages and risks of NIPT?

'The concept of screening is not intuitive and not everyone understands or thinks about it. So it [cffDNA] might be seen as diagnostic, when it is rarely so.' 'People do not have to think about non-invasive tests deeply, as they might be seen as just another blood test in pregnancy. They remove the "ethical step" of risk of pregnancy loss, which forces prospective parents to decide on whether they want this information at all, and what they might do with it—for example, would they consider selective termination?'

NIPT and NIPD were introduced in the NHS to detect Down syndrome and serious single gene disorders; what about other applications of the technology?

'cffDNA tests can be straightforwardly extended to more conditions, even up to whole genome sequencing. So there can be "mission creep", especially as commercial providers have every interest in having their technologies used more and more to derive more profit.

Because the "ethical step" (explained above) is removed, cffDNA tests will be used by the vast majority of prospective parents. This means a higher proportion of pregnancies affected by disabilities such as Down syndrome will potentially be identified. This could lead to the elimination of Down syndrome and ultimately many other conditions, via an increase in the number of abortions. As cffDNA testing is extended, the line between "serious condition" and "minor difference" is eroded.'

In Tom's introduction to this report on the ethics of genetic testing, he stresses the importance of consultation and learning about the rich and varied lives of disabled people rather than just focusing on mutations or genetic spelling mistakes. If people are to make free choices for their families, Tom reminds us that we also need confidence that our society will welcome disabled children, and support them and their families appropriately.

  Tasks and Discussion Points

Review the information provided on the NHS website about NIPT services: www.rapid.nhs.uk/guides-to-nipd-nipt

Discuss its applications and the pros and cons of using this technology.

Key Points

- Screening is used to identify individuals with an increased risk of having a condition.
- A diagnostic test is used confirm a diagnosis.
- NIPT to screen for trisomy and Down syndrome, is not a definitive diagnostic test, and an invasive diagnostic test (using chorionic villus sampling or amniocentesis) is used to confirm an abnormal result from NIPT.

Liquid Biopsy and Oncology

The technical success of NIPT and NGS for the analysis of cell-free circulating DNA has encouraged the development of similar *liquid biopsy* strategies for cancer patients with solid tumours such as breast cancer or colorectal cancer. Somatic mutations that drive the development of cancers or which result in drug resistance can be detected using NGS. The use of liquid biopsy (taking a blood sample for the analysis of cell-free tumour DNA) has potential advantages from a patient safety perspective, because taking serial biopsies from multiple tissues from cancer patients who are undergoing treatment can result in infection and other complications. This strategy may also be more valid scientifically because tumours evolve over time and are genetically heterogeneous; liquid biopsy may give the oncologist a clearer snapshot of the important genetic targets for treatment at particular time-points over the course of the patient's disease. The clinical utility and the health economics of such a personalized approach in oncology care is the subject of ongoing research.

3.7   Screening and NGS: the Clinical, Social, and Ethical Considerations

In theory, NGS could be used in population screening to contribute to disease prevention, through risk prediction and mitigation. As the costs of sequencing have declined, the notion of sequencing the genomes of healthy individuals has gained support. If this were carried out from birth (as part of existing new-born-screening initiatives), we could envisage a transcript of NGS data like a *DNA passport* to supplement the other data in our medical records, and that is reviewed throughout our lifetimes.

However, there are risks to be considered for using WGS and WES in non-symptomatic individuals. There is a significant risk of over-diagnosis of disease by generating false-positive results (by interpreting benign genetic variants as pathogenic) and because of incomplete penetrance. Over-diagnosis is problematic because it results in over-treatment, with inevitable side-effects and complications; and it also causes psychological harm, through anxiety and stigma.

> In Chapters 4 and 5 there are examples of known pathogenic variants that do not result in disease for all individuals.

There are several models for the use of WGS data. The bioinformatics linked to data from NGS could certainly be used for whole genome analysis from birth but the usefulness of this may be questionable because of the VUS discussed earlier. The data could therefore be subjected to selected analyses. Perhaps only genes known to be mutated in human diseases could be analysed or access to the data could be linked to specific episodes of illness? For example searching for functional variants of the *CFTR* gene for individuals who are symptomatic for cystic fibrosis, or the analysis of the relevant genes for a drug pathway if we want to predict response to a particular medicine.

Selected genome analysis and a focus on *gene panels* would avoid the need for the patient or their doctor to grapple with incidental findings and unsolicited information. Studies show that most of us want to receive all of the genetic information relevant to us if we have WGS and WES tests. However, there is a psychological and social impact of being told about unexpected inherited risk factors; in particular when we consider diseases for which there are no preventive and few therapeutic options, for example, dementia.

≋ Chapter Summary

- Molecular genetic laboratory methods from PCR to NGS have been developed and adapted to provide diagnostic and screening tests for specialized genetic services.
- Screening is used to identify individuals with an increased risk of having a condition. A diagnostic test is used confirm a diagnosis.
- NGS has proven itself as a landmark technology because it combines the precision and resolution of molecular diagnostics with the genome-wide perspective of classical cytogenetics.

- WGS and WES are applied to the diagnosis of rare diseases.
- Bioinformatics is an emerging clinical science that has developed alongside the use of whole genome analysis. Bioinformatic pipelines are used to filter genomic data; and to separate candidate pathogenic variants from benign variants and those of unknown significance.
- The sensitivity of molecular diagnostic strategies such as the detection of cffDNA and circulating tumour DNA has resulted in minimally invasive sampling protocols for use in prenatal testing and oncology services.
- Medical policy, and legal and ethical frameworks for the use of genetic testing, should be discussed and reviewed by the widest possible community, to consider the clinical value and acceptability of genome analysis.

Discussion Questions

3.1 Read this review and list some clinical applications for next generation sequencing: Ashley, E.A. (2016). Towards precision medicine. *Nature Reviews Genetics* 17(9), 507–22. doi:10.1038/nrg.2016.86

3.2 Read section 3.1 of this chapter and explain or discuss the significance of PCR as a laboratory technique.

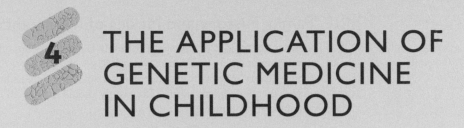

4 THE APPLICATION OF GENETIC MEDICINE IN CHILDHOOD

Learning Objectives

By the end of this chapter, you should be able to:

- explain how patients and families with genetic disorders are identified and how genetic data (including family history) is used;

- compare modes of inheritance and the underlying mutations associated with single gene disorders;

- explain aneuploidy and structural chromosomal rearrangements;

- distinguish predictive and diagnostic testing and explain the application of clinical and ethical guidelines to **genetic counselling**.

The burden of genetic disease in childhood is high. Most obviously for the child and their family, but also for society. Although individually rare, collectively genetic diseases account for a high proportion of death and disability, particularly in infancy. Occasionally, diseases may manifest as regressive conditions, with progressive loss of skills and functions, usually culminating in early death.

Genetic disorders are diagnosed:

- during pregnancy or at birth (**congenital abnormalities**);

- from screening of the newborn;

- in early life with developmental delay;

- and in the older child with learning difficulties; or with abnormal growth or puberty.

Genetic disorders are traditionally classified as chromosomal disorders, monogenic (Mendelian) disorders, or polygenic disorders, the latter of which will be considered in Chapters 5 and 6. Classification and diagnosis relies on an understanding of modes of inheritance, coupled with information from a detailed family history and physical examination. Sometimes the diagnosis is clinically evident from examination alone, as in the chromosomal disorder, Down syndrome. However, even in this situation, an understanding of the genetic cause is crucial to proper counselling of the family.

Genetic testing needs to take place within a robust ethical framework and requires careful consideration of why the test is being done and the potential ramifications of a positive test. Proper counselling of the family will include consideration of the scope of the test, and the potential to identify incidental findings. This is particularly relevant to whole exome sequencing (WES), where all known coding DNA is sequenced.

4.1   Family History and Modes of Inheritance

❯ The concept of the family history was introduced in the Bigger Picture Panel 2.1 in Chapter 2

We will consider this topic in depth here. The family history is an important tool for the recognition and classification of a possible genetic disorder. Enquiring into the family history may be a sensitive issue for some individuals and needs to be done with tact and understanding. The history should include all information known about the following:

- parents, siblings and half-siblings, grandparents, aunts, uncles, and cousins;
- any deaths, including the age and cause of death and associated health conditions;
- any family history of learning problems or developmental delay;
- any history of miscarriages and stillbirths;
- any consanguinity (by simply asking, are you and your partner related?).

The family tree is conventionally recorded using a pedigree diagram. The pedigree diagram is a very succinct way of presenting complex information. It may be embellished with social information, appropriate to the clinical case and the diagnoses under consideration.

❯ and that are also illustrated in the Bigger Picture Panel 2.1

When drawing the pedigree, there are certain conventions that are useful to observe, Review Figure 4.1, and Case Studies 4.1 and 4.2, which illustrate these conventions.

Patterns, or modes, of inheritance are often associated with particular disease phenotypes. However, an inheritance pattern will depend on the chromosome locus and the impact of the particular allele or alleles that underlie the trait. Some diseases show locus heterogeneity too, because they can be caused by mutations in a number of genes. Therefore, for a given disease phenotype it is possible to observe more than one associated pattern of inheritance.

When evaluating a pedigree diagram, it is important to consider three key issues: *transmission* of the condition from one generation to the next, the *sex-ratio* of affected individuals, and the pattern of *segregation* of the condition within the family. Tentative inferences can then be made about the mode of inheritance of the disease. For example:

- Transmission

  For example, if affected individuals of both sexes are found in multiple generations, this suggests a dominant inheritance pattern.

  Sporadic genetic disease may be due to chromosomal abnormalities, recessive inheritance, or because of new (*de novo*) deleterious mutations in a single locus.

- Sex-ratios

  For example, X-linked inheritance is unlikely if equal numbers of males and females are affected.

- Segregation

  For example, if the disease is transmitting via unaffected females, this suggests X-linked recessive inheritance. If all children of affected mothers are also affected, and there are no affected children from affected fathers, mitochondrial inheritance should be considered.

Figure 4.1 Family history (pedigree diagram). The conventions for recording a family history are indicated in this diagram. There is a set of agreed symbols to use when drawing a pedigree. In order to show how individuals are related to each other, lines are drawn between symbols. The correct placement of these lines is an important clinical skill to ensure the pedigree gives an accurate picture of family relationships.

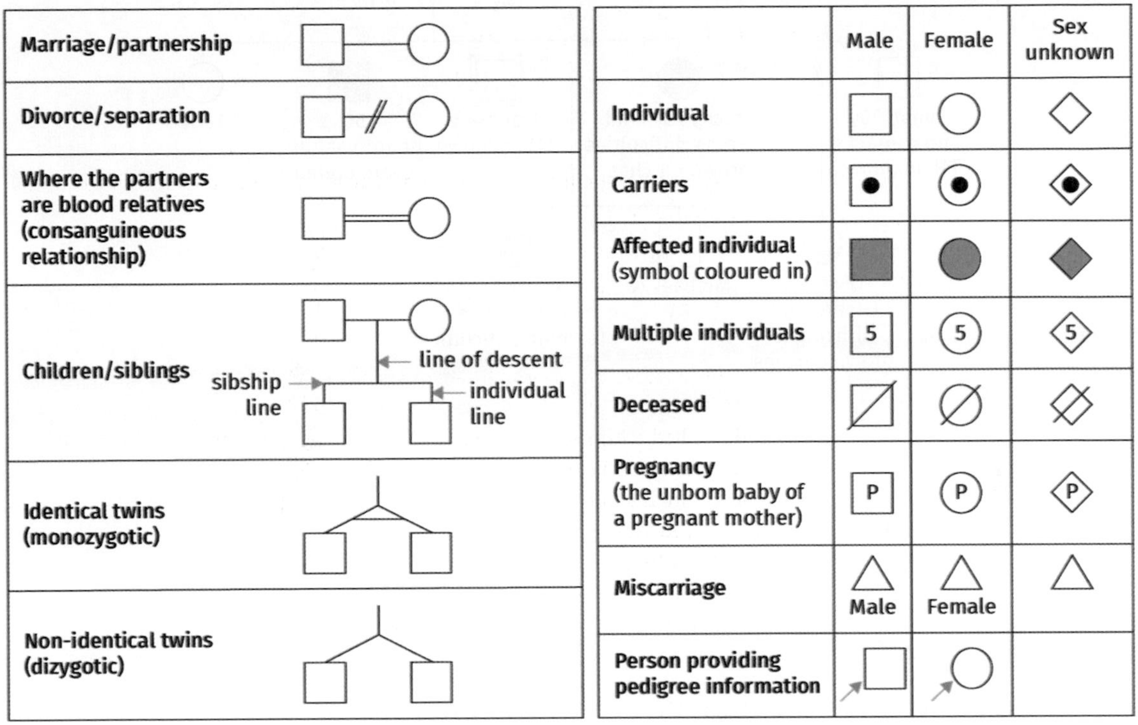

Illustration based on original ideas courtesy of Health Education England's Genomics Education Programme.

Case Study 4.1
Autosomal dominant (AD) inheritance—a family history

Stacey is concerned about her son, Frank Jr. Stacey has recently been diagnosed with neurofibromatosis after her ophthalmologist noted characteristic eye abnormalities.

Frank Jr has learning difficulties and hyperactivity. Stacey's oldest child, Evie, by a previous relationship, also has learning problems and, like Stacey, she has brown skin patches. Stacey's mother died of breast cancer at fifty-seven years of age, and Stacey thinks she also had brown patches. Stacey's father has glaucoma but is otherwise well. Stacey's uncle lives in a residential home for people with learning disabilities. He has a leg deformity

from a chronic non-healing fracture and neurodisability with severe epilepsy. Stacey's partner is well but was adopted at birth and his family history is unknown.

The history suggests multiple family members were affected with neurofibromatosis Type 1, an autosomal dominant condition. This pattern of inheritance is indicated by apparent vertical transmission through three generations, affecting males and females. The brown patches, known as café-au-lait patches, learning difficulties, behaviour problems, neurodisability, non-healing fractures and breast cancer are all recognized features of neurofibromatosis.

Figure 4.2 The family history described in a pedigree diagram.

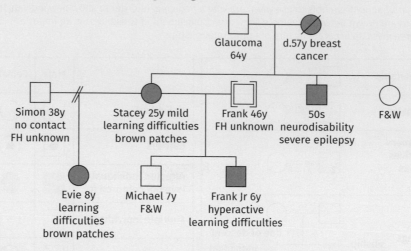

Glaucoma
64y

d.57y breast
cancer

Simon 38y
no contact
FH unknown

Stacey 25y mild
learning difficulties
brown patches

Frank 46y
FH unknown

50s
neurodisability
severe epilepsy

F&W

Evie 8y
learning
difficulties
brown patches

Michael 7y
F&W

Frank Jr 6y
hyperactive
learning difficulties

Case Study 4.2
Autosomal recessive (AR) inheritance—a family history

The proband indicated with the arrow had ambiguous genitalia at birth, secondary to **Congenital Adrenal Hyperplasia** (CAH). This is one of the commonest causes of disorders of sex development in females. Her older brother was known to be affected by CAH, as was her maternal cousin.

Figure 4.3 The family history is illustrated in the pedigree diagram.

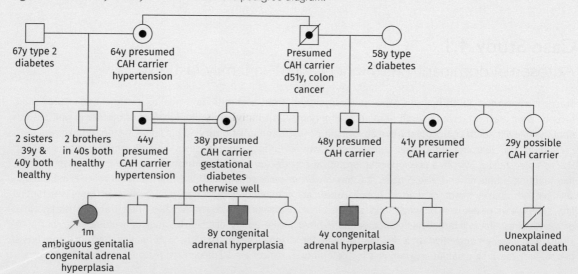

67y type 2
diabetes

64y presumed
CAH carrier
hypertension

Presumed
CAH carrier
d51y, colon
cancer

58y type
2 diabetes

2 sisters
39y &
40y both
healthy

2 brothers
in 40s both
healthy

44y
presumed
CAH carrier
hypertension

38y presumed
CAH carrier
gestational
diabetes
otherwise well

48y presumed
CAH carrier

41y presumed
CAH carrier

29y possible
CAH carrier

1m
ambiguous genitalia
congenital adrenal
hyperplasia

8y congenital
adrenal hyperplasia

4y congenital
adrenal hyperplasia

Unexplained
neonatal death

Another male cousin had died unexpectedly at ten days old, but the cause was unknown, but this may well have been due to unrecognized metabolic problems because of CAH. Her parents were first cousins; her paternal grandmother and maternal grandfather were siblings.

CAH may pass unnoticed in boys, but in girls leads to virilization of the genitalia, which appear abnormal at birth.

By inference, it is possible to deduce the carrier status of parents and grandparents. This family history demonstrates **consanguinity**.

Notice that all individuals affected by this condition are recorded in one generation of the pedigree diagram. This horizontal pattern of transmission is typical of an AR condition.

Key Points

- Standard notation is used by clinicians to describe the family history of genetic conditions and other traits.
- Taking a family history is important for determining the mode of inheritance of a particular trait and to guide genetic counselling. Drawing and reviewing a pedigree diagram can help with this.

4.2   Introducing Monogenic Disorders and Mendelian Inheritance

If a mutation in a single gene is sufficient and necessary to cause a phenotype we describe the trait as monogenic. We often see characteristic patterns of inheritance for monogenic traits based on predictions made by Gregor Mendel, which is why the terms *monogenic* and *Mendelian* are often used interchangeably.

In classical Mendelian inheritance, traits are described as recessive or dominant. Their classification also depends on the locus of the mutated gene (does it lie on an autosome or on one of the sex chromosomes?). Some well-known monogenic traits are unrelated to disease, such as those for eye colour and some blood groups. However, there are also several thousand individual monogenic diseases described in the curated catalogue *Online Mendelian Inheritance in Man* (OMIM).

If a mutation in one copy of a single autosomal gene is sufficient to produce a phenotype or disease, then the trait or condition is described as autosomal dominant (AD). The phenotype is observed in heterozygotes, who only carry one mutated allele and a 'normal' allele.

When the unaffected (wild type) allele on an autosome can compensate for the effect of the mutated allele in heterozygotes, the associated traits are described as autosomal recessive (AR). For disease to result there must be inheritance of two copies of the mutated gene. The trait can be expressed in individuals who are homozygous for the same pathogenic mutation and in compound heterozygotes for two different pathogenic variants, i.e. the mutations need not be identical. In most instances, both parents would be carriers, but occasionally, one of the mutant alleles arises as a new mutation (*de novo* mutation), which is significant for counselling parents about risks of further affected children.

Sex-linked monogenic inheritance results from the mutation of genes on the X chromosome. As males only have one X chromosome, they are described as hemizygous for mutant alleles. X-linked mutations can cause recessive and dominant traits.

> For example. the *HFE* mutations that cause Type 1 Hereditary Haemochromatosis are very common in European populations and are discussed in Chapter 5.

Autosomal Recessive (AR) Inheritance

Diseases inherited in an AR pattern are typically severe, and are rare. Examples include cystic fibrosis, sickle cell disease, and phenylketonuria. Further children from the same relationship may be affected but a prior family history would be very unusual, unless there is significant consanguinity in the family history, or a very high carrier frequency in a particular population. See Case Study 4.2, which illustrates a horizontal pattern of transmission, which means all affected individuals are observed in one generation, and is a characteristic transmission pattern for AR conditions.

In some populations, such as in Japan, the Indian subcontinent and the Middle East, consanguineous relationships are common; with the great majority of such relationships being first-cousin unions. Similarly, in genetically isolated populations such as island communities, or those separated by religion, culture, or language, otherwise rare mutations are found at a much higher frequency. Consequently, certain conditions are much more common in these isolated populations than in the wider population. For example, some western Pacific Island populations have a high prevalence (5 per cent) of achromatopsia, which is a very rare form of colour blindness and poor vision (the worldwide prevalence is only ~ 0.003 per cent).

Another example of AR traits with high carrier frequencies is where the heterozygous state confers a survival benefit. An example of heterozygote advantage is the presence of high carrier frequencies for the mutations that cause sickle-cell disease in malaria-endemic regions, such as Africa and the Mediterranean. This is now thought to be because the underlying mutation interferes with the replication of the malarial parasite in the red blood cells of individuals who carry the mutation.

In populations susceptible to particular AR conditions, neonatal screening is often instituted to allow timely intervention and effective treatment at an early stage. In the UK, only nine genetic conditions are screened for at birth as of 2018 (see Table 4.1).

Table 4.1 AR conditions screened for at birth as part of the UK National Neonatal Screening Programme.

AR Disease	OMIM Number
Phenylketonuria	#261600
Hypothyroidism (15 % cases are AR)	#218700 & #275200
Sickle Cell disease	#603903
Cystic Fibrosis	#219700
Medium Chain Acyl-CoA Dehydrogenase Deficiency	#201450
Maple Syrup Urine Disease	#248600
Isovaleric Acidemia	#243500
Glutaric Aciduria Type 1	#231670
Homocystinuria	#236200

Online Mendelian Inheritance in Man (OMIM) is a database of all Mendelian disorders. It describes about 4,000 individual diseases. Each OMIM entry has its own specific number linked to a disease and associated gene variants. Standard nomenclature is used that is congruent with that used by the Human Genome Organisation. The number of each disease description in the OMIM catalogue is listed in column 2.

Autosomal Dominant (AD) Inheritance

AD conditions often affect successive generations of a family because a single pathogenic autosomal allele is sufficient to produce the disease phenotype. Figure 4.2 illustrates the typical vertical pattern of transmission. However, these conditions often arise *de novo* too, with no previous family history. For example, 80 per cent of cases of achondroplasia arise from new mutations. The likelihood of recurrence for siblings is negligible, but any children of the affected individual will have a 1:2, or 50 per cent chance of being affected.

Three principal mutational mechanisms that were explained in Chapter 2 underlie most AD diseases. These are loss of function mutations (and haploinsufficiency), dominant negative mutations, and gain of function mutations.

Achondroplasia is an abnormality of skeletal tissue that leads to short stature with a distinctive appearance. It is caused by gain of function mutations in the *FGFR3* gene, resulting in over-activity of the protein Fibroblast Growth Factor Receptor 3 and impaired cartilage and bone formation. Table 4.2 provides further examples of mutations that cause AD conditions.

Modifiers of Phenotype: Penetrance and Expressivity

Although a genetic disorder may be caused by a particular genotype (for a single locus), the phenotype that we observe results from a complex set of interactions between that genotype, other modifying genes, and the environment.

Penetrance describes the proportion of individuals who express the phenotype associated with a genotype. We see a marked variability in penetrance for some genotypes, and this may lead to generations being 'skipped' within a pedigree diagram. This may occur in conditions like neurofibromatosis that are also inherently variable in the expression of the disease for the individual. Individual variability in the expression of a disease with respect to severity or particular pathology is called expressivity.

> ❯ These concepts are considered in more depth, with examples in Chapter 5.

Triplet Repeat Disorders and Anticipation

Some monogenic disorders exhibit the phenomenon of anticipation. Anticipation refers to the increasing severity of a condition, and its occurrence at an earlier age of onset with successive generations. Anticipation is seen in a range of neurological conditions referred to as *trinucleotide repeat disorders*, caused by mutations that result in an expansion of a short (three nucleotide) tandem repeat.

Table 4.2 Mutations that cause AD conditions.

AD Disease	Gene Locus and Class of Mutation
Achondroplasia	*FGFR3*, GOF
Familial Hypercholesterolaemia	*LDLR*, LOF
Marfan Syndrome	*FBN1*, DN
Neurofibromatosis	*NF1*, LOF
Osteogenesis Imperfecta	COL1A1, DN

DN; dominant negative mutation, GOF; gain of function mutation, LOF; loss of function mutation.

More than twenty trinucleotide repeat disorders are known, all having a neu-rological phenotype, with most being AD. Trinucleotide repeats are susceptible to dynamic mutations in meiosis, with the resultant germ cells containing an expanded number of repeats compared with somatic cells.

The repetitive sequences that are expanded can occur in the coding regions or in the regulatory domains of the gene sequence. In *myotonic dystrophy*, a progressive neuromuscular disease, the 3' Untranslated Region (UTR) of the *DPMK* gene is expanded beyond its normal five to thirty repeats. A minor phe-notype is seen with over fifty repeats, overt disease is seen with over one hun-dred repeats, and a severe congenital form is seen with over 1,000 repeats. In myotonic dystrophy, the expansion occurs with maternal transmission—thus a mother—perhaps minimally affected at the time of giving birth—may have a severely affected infant with congenital myotonic dystrophy. The expansion of the UTR in myotonic dystrophy appears to reduce the expression of a number of genes in a dominant-negative manner.

In **Huntington's disease**, a severe neurodegenerative disorder, the normal (wild-type) gene encodes the Huntingtin (HTT) protein with a polyglutamine chain of six to thirty-five glutamine residues at its amino terminus. Disease results with more than forty glutamine residues, through a toxic gain of function in the resultant mutant Huntingtin protein (mHTT). Anticipation is more pronounced in fathers who have inherited the mutant gene from their mother—perhaps due to sex-specific epigenetic changes. Severe cases mani-fest in childhood, known as Juvenile Huntington's Disease, with onset before ten years of age.

> The penetrance of *HTT* mutations and adult onset HD are considered at the beginning of Chapter 5.

Sex-Linked Monogenic Inheritance

The Y chromosome is one of the two sex chromosomes and is the smallest chro-mosome in the human karyotype. It only bears a small number of genes, largely responsible for sex-determination (e.g. *SRY*) and spermatogenesis. In theory Y-linked disease should be recognizable from the male to male transmission pattern (holandric inheritance), because fathers pass their Y chromosome to their sons. However, very few pedigrees exhibiting Y-linked monogenic inher-itance have been described because mutations in genes involved in spermato-genesis affect fertility. There have been some recent rare reports of Y-linked hereditary hearing loss.

Sex-linked inheritance therefore results, almost exclusively, from expression of genes on the X chromosome. Affected genes on the X chromosome may be recessive or dominant. Recessive genes, such as those for haemophilia A, are usually silent in female carriers because the normal gene on one of the X chromosomes can compensate for the mutation on the other. Exceptionally, skewed X chromosome inactivation (XCI) may produce a disease phenotype in females. Read Bigger Picture Panel 4.1, for a discussion of the molecular basis of X-linked recessive inheritance and XCI.

X-linked recessive traits may be difficult to trace back through families, be-cause they may skip generations, through female carriers. The following fea-tures are observed in the family history of someone with an X-linked recessive trait; only males are affected; female carriers are unaffected; affected males never have affected sons (to whom they transmit their Y chromosome) but all daughters are obligate carriers and so can transmit the mutation.

Some X-linked recessive conditions, such as Duchenne Muscular Dystrophy, are of such severity that affected males do not have children, due to progressive and severe disability. Please see Case Study 4.3 for an example of a complex case study of family affected by Duchenne Muscular Dystrophy.

X-linked dominant disorders do affect females, but are usually more severe in males, as in the case of Fragile X syndrome, which is a leading cause of intellectual disability in males; and Alport syndrome, which causes the progressive kidney condition, glomerulonephritis. Some deleterious mutations for X-linked dominant conditions, appear to be lethal in the hemizygous state, thus sufferers are almost exclusively female (e.g. some *MEPC2* variants that cause the neuro-degenerative condition, Rett syndrome).

Historically, it has long been noted that there is a relative excess of males with intellectual disability. Fragile X syndrome is the most frequent cause of X-Linked intellectual disability (XLID) and is another example of a trinucleotide repeat disease. It is caused by a dynamic mutation that creates a fragile site on the X chromosome. The mutation occurs at maternal meiosis, and results in an expansion of a CGG triplet sequence in the 5' UTR, upstream of the gene *FMR1*.

❯ which is described in Table 4.5.

Bigger Picture Panel 4.1

The molecular basis of X-linked recessive inheritance and X Chromosome Inactivation (XCI)

Males (XY) are hemizygous for loci on the X chromosome because they have only one X chromosome. Males therefore express most X-linked recessive traits because they have no homologous normal/wild-type allele to compensate.

In females, one X chromosome is inactivated by epigenetic silencing, occurring at around fifteen or sixteen days post conception, when the embryo consists of some 5,000 cells. Thereafter, the inactivated X is passed on through successive generations of daughter cells; i.e. this epigenetic silencing is heritable in somatic cells. The inactivated X chromosome is visible in chromosome preparations in interphase cells as a Barr Body—a dark mass of chromatin. In men or women with multiple copies of the X chromosome, multiple Barr Bodies are visible.

The process of *X Chromosome Inactivation* (XCI) is often referred to as Lyonization, after the Norwich-born geneticist Dr Mary Lyon, who first proposed the concept in 1961. XCI is dependent on the *XIST* gene located on the long arm of the inactivated X chromosome. Silencing of the expression of the inactivated genes is achieved by DNA methylation.

Inactivation of either the maternally or paternally inherited X chromosome is usually random; but if it is skewed, female expression of some X-linked recessive disorders can occur. The random pattern of X inactivation, and consequently gene expression, is responsible for variation in coat colour in cats and a similar phenomenon may be seen in women with pigmentary disorders.

The process of XCI ensures that males and females have essentially the same dosage and expression level for X-linked genes. However, the tips of the X-chromosomes, the so-called *pseudoautosomal regions* (PAR1 & 2) are not inactivated. PAR1 contains the key growth gene, *SHOX* (Short Stature Homeobox Gene), which is also found on the Y chromosome. The loss of one copy of *SHOX* is the major contributor to the short stature seen in Turner syndrome which is described in Table 4.5.

XCI is a variable phenomenon, with considerable disparity between cells, consequently some genes on the X chromosome, in addition to *XIST* and *SHOX*, are active.

Mitochondrial Inheritance and Heteroplasmy

Every cell contains thousands of mitochondria. These organelles are fundamental for a range of metabolic functions. Mitochondria have their own DNA and are almost entirely inherited from the oocyte. Thus, mitochondrial disease has a unique pattern of **matrilineal inheritance**. Mitochondrial diseases are passed from a mother to all her children, (subject to variable expressivity) whereas affected males *never* have affected children because the mitochondria are almost exclusively transmitted via the oocyte, not the spermatozoa. See Figure 4.4 for an illustration of mitochondrial inheritance within a family.

This unique pattern means that mitochondrial inheritance can be distinguished from simple AD inheritance.

The mitochondrial genome is relatively small and encodes ribosomal RNA production and transfer RNAs required for mitochondrial protein synthesis and some of the proteins involved in oxidative phosphorylation. Mitochondrial diseases are most often manifest in the brain, heart, and muscle. Other associated conditions may include diabetes and renal disease. See Table 4.3 for a summary of recognized mitochondrial disease phenotypes.

Mitochondria are randomly distributed to daughter cells. All mitochondria within a cell can be identical (entirely wild type for a particular locus or entirely mutant), a single population of genetically identical mitochondria is referred to as homoplasmy. If a cell contains a mixed population of mitochondria, some with a mutation, and others without; this is called **heteroplasmy**. Heteroplasmy results in variable expression of mitochondrial diseases. The distribution of mutant mitochondria may differ in different tissues resulting in a highly variable phenotype, even with the same underlying genetic mutation.

The phenomenon of heteroplasmy makes prenatal diagnosis of mitochondrial disease very challenging. In order to overcome this, the UK Human Fertilisation & Embryology Authority recently approved the creation of what the popular press has dubbed '*three parent*' babies.

Figure 4.4 A pedigree diagram from a family affected by mitochondrial deafness. Matrilineal inheritance is demonstrated, although subject III.7 appears unaffected, reflecting the variable phenotype of mitochondrial disease.

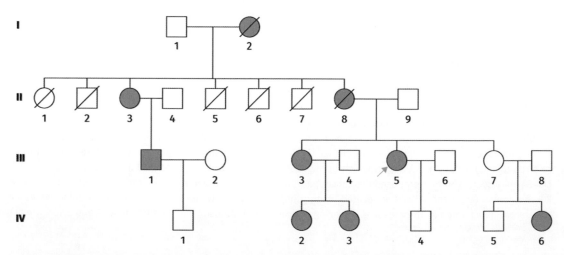

Adapted from Mutai, H., Watabe, T., Kosaki, K., Ogawa, K., and Matsunaga, T. (2017). Mitochondrial mutations in maternally inherited hearing loss. *BMC Medical Genetics*, 18(1), [32]. doi:10.1186/s12881-017-0389-4, with permission.

Table 4.3 Summary of recognized mitochondrial disease phenotypes. The site of the mitochondrial mutation is often described with the abbreviation m., followed by the nucleotide position.

Disorder	Description
MERRF (Myoclonic Epilepsy & Ragged Red Fibres)	Progressive myoclonic epilepsy, myopathy (with classic appearance on microscopy using Gomori's trichrome staining), encephalopathy and dementia. Optic atrophy is usually present. Caused by mutations in lysine tRNA.
MELAS (Myoclonic Epilepsy, Lactic Acidosis and Stroke-like episodes)	The hallmark of the condition is stroke-like episodes, often with headache, hemianopia (loss of half the visual field) and hemiplegia. Epilepsy, sensorineural hearing loss, short stature and diabetes also occur commonly. A number of mutations may give this phenotype (**genocopies**).
NARP (Neurodegeneration, Ataxia and Retinitis Pigmentosa)	Caused by a mutation in m.8993 (the 'NARP mutation'), the main early symptom is night blindness. Epilepsy may occur at any stage. Neurodegeneration and dementia occurs in older adults.
Leigh's Disease	Leigh's disease is a severe neurodegenerative disease of early onset, and usually culminates in early death. It may arise from mitochondrial, AR (*SURF1*) and X-linked (*NDUFA1*) mutations affecting cytochrome C, a crucial complex in oxidative phosphorylation.
Leber's Hereditary Optic Neuropathy (LHON)	Leber's typically presents with painless central visual loss in young adults (18–30 years). Males are affected much more commonly. 70% are due to the mutation m.11778, although 18 mutations are known.
Mitochondrial Deafness	Mitochondrial DNA mutations m.1555A > G and m.3243A > G are the primary causes of mitochondrial sensorineural hearing loss. The usual phenotype is progressive hearing loss in adult life, but patients are extremely sensitive to ototoxic antibiotics called aminoglycosides, such as gentamicin, when even a single dose may produce profound hearing loss.
Kearns–Sayre Syndrome	Kearns–Sayre syndrome is mainly characterized by somatic mutation in the mitochondrial genome, including large deletions of many genes that are essential to mitochondrial function. The syndrome results in ophthalmoparesis and retinitis pigmentosa in childhood, associated with neurological features (ataxia and proximal myopathy), cardiac conduction block, short stature and often, multiple endocrinopathies including diabetes, hypoparathyroidism, and adrenal insufficiency.

The methods used result in an egg with nuclear DNA from the mother, and mitochondrial DNA from a donor; which is then fertilized with the father's sperm. It allows the donor's healthy mitochondria to replace the mitochondria with the maternal mutations. The first 'three-parent' child born by these techniques was reported in April 2016, to a mother whose two previous children had died of the mitochondrial disorder, Leigh's disease.

❯ which is a condition described in Table 4.3.

 Key Points

- Some curious features of monogenic inheritance are because of the phenomena: variable penetrance, variable expressivity, anticipation, and mitochondrial inheritance.

Figure 4.5 One example of *three parent* IVF, which can be used to prevent mitochondrial disorders.

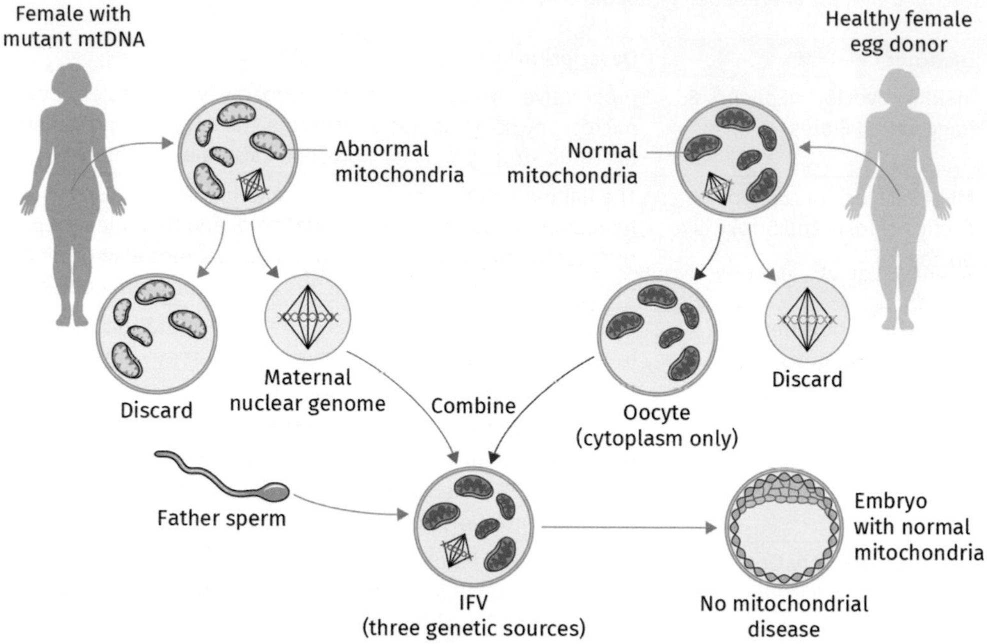

Reprinted by permission from Springer Nature. Tanaka, A. J., Sauer, M. V., Egli, D., and Kort, D. H. (2013). Harnessing the stem cell potential: the path to prevent mitochondrial disease. *Nature Medicine*, 19, 1578–9. Copyright © 2013, Springer Nature.

4.3 Chromosomal Disorders

Chromosomal abnormalities are common, affecting ~ 1 per cent of live births, 5 per cent of stillborn infants, and 50 per cent of first trimester miscarriages. A normal diploid cell has twenty-three pairs of chromosomes: forty-four autosomes and two sex chromosomes (XX or XY) and there are notable examples of disorders that affect the autosomes and the sex chromosomes. Chromosome abnormalities can change the dosage and organization of many genes simultaneously. The underlying mutation can result in numerical or structural changes that can be classified as described in Table 4.4. Many possible chromosomal aberrations that arise at meiosis are lethal *in utero*, or are not compatible with life soon after birth.

Table 4.4 Classifying chromosome abnormalities.

Numerical	Structural	Mixoploidy
Aneuploidy, e.g. trisomy and monosomy	Reciprocal translocation	Mosaicism
Polyploidy, e.g. triploidy and tetraploidy	Robertsonian translocation	Chimerism
	Deletion	
	Inversion	
	Isochromosome	
	Ring chromosome	

Individuals with a chromosome abnormality may have mixed cell lines (mixoploidy), which has two possible causes. Mosaicism is the presence of two or more cell lines derived from a single zygote because of a mutation arising during mitosis in early embryogenesis; and chimerism is two or more distinct cell lines that are of different genetic origin because they are derived from more than one zygote.

The conditions arising from chromosome abnormalities result from gene dosage effects (over-expression of genes and haploinsufficiency); and/or by the gross rearrangement of genetic loci, resulting in aberrant regulation of gene expression.

Aneuploidy

An abnormal chromosome number is the most common congenital chromosomal abnormality. Aneuploidy is the loss or gain of one or more whole chromosomes; for example resulting in a monosomy or trisomy. These abnormalities are usually caused by the failure of homologous chromosomes to separate (non-disjunction) during meiosis, or by the loss of a chromosome as it moves to the pole of cell (anaphase-lag) during meiosis.

Numerical disorders are described according to their abnormal karyotype, referring to the total number of chromosomes; plus or minus the altered chromosome number. See Table 4.5 describing some syndromes associated with particular aneuploidies, and the karyotype associated with trisomy 21 is illustrated in Figure 4.6.

Figure 4.6 Down syndrome human karyotype 47,XY,+21. Trisomy 21 (Down syndrome) associated male karyotype; 47,XY,+21. This individual has a full chromosome complement plus an extra chromosome 21.

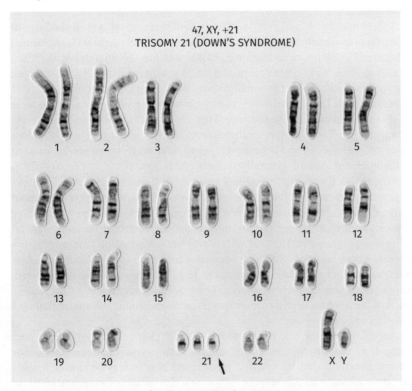

Table 4.5 Aneuploidies associated with recurrent chromosomal disorders and the nomenclature used to describe the karyotype.

Aneuploidy	International Standard Chromosome Nomenclature	Syndrome
Trisomy 21	47,XX,+21 or 47,XY,+21	Down syndrome
Trisomy 18	47,XX,+18 or 47,XY,+18	Edwards syndrome
Trisomy 13	47,XX,+13 or 47,XY,+13	Patau syndrome
45,X*	45,X0	Turner syndrome
47,XXY	47,XXY	Klinefelter syndrome

*Monosomy of X is the only viable monosomy in humans.

The term syndrome can be defined as a group of signs and symptoms that occur together in a condition or disease as described for the example of Turner syndrome with Table 4.6. The association of a wide range of pathologies and other traits with in chromosome abnormalities is caused by the multiple gene loci that are affected. Genetic syndromes are often named after the person who first described them in the medical literature, but more recently names are used that describe the symptoms or the underlying genetic etiology. For example, Down syndrome is now often referred to as trisomy 21.

Down syndrome arises from the classical trisomy in about 95 per cent of cases, mostly arising from non-disjunction in maternal meiosis I. It affects around 1:1,000 pregnancies in the UK and the incidence rises with maternal age; with one in one hundred pregnancies affected in mothers aged forty, for example.

Approximately 4 per cent of Down syndrome cases are secondary to Robertsonian translocations, a condition described in 'Structural Chromosomal Abnormalities' later in this chapter. Mosaicism for the underlying mutation occurs in about 1 per cent of cases, and this is associated with a less severe phenotype; and in this case, the condition may not be recognized at birth.

Infants with Down syndrome typically have low birth weight, low muscle tone, and a typical facial appearance. They are also at risk of a range of serious congenital cardiac and other malformations, such as bowel problems. Children have delayed growth and neurodevelopment with moderate to severe learning difficulties, but they are generally sociable and happy.

Trisomy 13 (Patau syndrome) and trisomy 18 (Edwards syndrome) are exceptionally severe conditions, often complicated by multiple severe congenital anomalies of the brain, heart, gut and other organs. They each have a distinctive phenotype, are very rare; and are most commonly detected through prenatal screening programmes. The prognosis is very limited, although longer-term survival has been reported with more aggressive medical intervention. Prognosis is somewhat better in mosaic and partial forms. If trisomy 18 or 13 is suspected, urgent molecular cytogenetic analysis is needed to guide treatment decisions—such as the need for urgent cardiac surgery, or to determine the appropriateness of ongoing intensive care.

Aneuploidy of the sex chromosomes (X and Y) is relatively common and arises from non-disjunction, during meiosis or in the early embryo. The loss or gain of genetic material may affect all daughter cells or may be partial, leading to tissue mosaicism. Aneuploidy of the sex chromosomes may not result in

Table 4.6 Clinical features observed in Turner syndrome.

Prenatal	- Increased nuchal translucency on antenatal fetal anomaly scan
	- Incidental finding on amniocentesis
Dysmorphic Features	- Congenital lymphedema
	- Short and/or webbed neck with low posterior hairline 30%
	- Widespread nipples & shield chest
	- Congenital hip dislocation
Dermatological	- Small, brittle hyperconvex nails
	- Increased melanocytic naevi
	- Keloid scarring
Congenital Heart Disease	- Coarctation of aorta
	- Bicuspid aortic valve
	- Hypoplastic left-heart syndrome
	- Dilatation of aortic root (adulthood)
Cognition	- Learning disabilities (nonverbal perceptual motor and visuospatial skills) (in 70%)
	- Developmental delay (in 10%)
	- Social awkwardness
Endocrine	- Short stature by age 5 (95%)
	- Increased carrying angle of elbow (cubitus valgus)
	- Madelung deformity (chondrodysplasia of distal radial epiphysis)
	- Autoimmune thyroid disease (30%)
Gastrointestinal	- Coeliac disease
	- Crohn's disease
Renal	- Horseshoe kidney
	- Wilm's tumour
Sensory	- Chronic Secretory Otitis Media ('Glue Ear♀')
	- Progressive sensorineural hearing loss (universal by age 40)
	- Ptosis (drooping of eyelids)
	- Strabismus ('Squint')
	- Cataracts
Adolescence	- Absent or arrested puberty secondary to gonadal failure (Gonadal Dysgenesis)
	- Gonadoblastoma
	- Scoliosis 10%
Adulthood	- Infertility
	- Osteoporosis
	- Hypertension
	- Type 2 Diabetes

abnormal physical characteristics (**dysmorphism**) at birth and may pass unnoticed unless called to attention by abnormal growth, delayed or absent puberty, infertility or other abnormalities.

Turner syndrome is seen in around 1 in 4,000 female live births, and arises from partial or complete monosomy of the X chromosome, usually arising from paternal meiosis (80 per cent). Studies have shown that the majority of Turner syndrome conceptions result in spontaneous miscarriage.

Structural chromosome abnormalities may also cause Turner syndrome, including ring chromosome formation or **isochromosome** of the X chromosome, which results from the loss of one arm of the X chromosome (most commonly p arm), with duplication of the other arm, with the karyotype denoted as 46,X,i(Xq). With some mutations, notably ring X chromosome variants, the crucial *XIST* gene is deleted, resulting in a markedly abnormal phenotype due to excess gene dosage effects, as XCI is reliant on this gene .

❯ see Bigger Picture Panel 4.1.

One possible complication of Turner syndrome is the potential for X-linked diseases to arise. In this situation, the subject has only one functional X chromosome. Cases of classical haemophilia, Duchenne muscular dystrophy and other X-linked conditions have been reported in association with Turner syndrome.

Klinefelter syndrome occurs in approximately 1 in 1,000 live male births and is associated with the karyotype 47,XXY in about 80 per cent of cases. Other karyotypes show mosaicism (46,XY/47,XXY) or an even higher X chromosome aneuploidy, such as 48,XXXY. Klinefelter syndrome is associated with a range of difficulties ranging from speech and language impairment in early life to hypogonadism and infertility in adult life. Intelligence is affected to a variable degree, but most boys are within the normal range. Early speech difficulties are linked to educational difficulties and impaired socialization, sometimes with autistic features. Although it usually starts at the normal time, progress through the milestones of puberty is slower, as hypogonadism results in lower testosterone levels. Phenotypically, boys with Klinefelter's are tall due to having an additional copy of the key growth gene, *SHOX*, found on both the X and Y chromosomes. The testes are small and infertile but with the use of modern fertility techniques fertility is possible. Gynaecomastia (male breast development) is common, affecting around 50 per cent, and there is an increased rate of breast cancer in adulthood, relative to unaffected males.

Structural Chromosomal Abnormalities

Structural chromosomal abnormalities arise from the breakage and joining of chromosomes to create a novel configuration. The rearrangements can involve one, two, or multiple chromosomes and can be balanced with no loss or gain of genetic material or unbalanced with insertions and deletions that affect gene dosage. See Figure 4.7 for illustrations of some structural chromosomal abnormalities that can arise.

A **reciprocal translocation** in which there is simply a change in the relative locations of genes on the rearranged chromosomes can affect any pair of chromosomes. A reciprocal translocation may not affect gene dosage or have any functional consequence, but if the breakpoints fall within a gene locus a translocation could disrupt gene expression. A Robertsonian translocation affects two of the **acrocentric chromosomes** (these are chromosomes 13, 14, 15, 21, and 22). For these chromosomes, the centromere is located near one end of the chromosome and their p arms are made up of repetitive

Figure 4.7 An illustration of structural chromosomal abnormalities. Chromosomal translocations affect around 1:600 liveborn infants. A translocation refers to the non-homologous recombination of part of one chromosome with another. Duplication or deletion at the site of recombination may occur, resulting in gene imbalance.

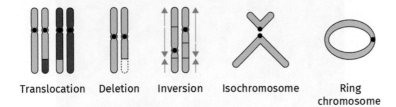

Translocation   Deletion   Inversion   Isochromosome   Ring chromosome

DNA sequences. These satellite DNA sequences can be lost in a Robertsonian translocation with no effect on phenotype; and when these **acrocentric chromosomes** are fused, the overall chromosome count will be forty-five instead of forty-six. However, when an individual who carries a Robertsonian translocation produces gametes, there is a risk that there will be loss or gain of genetic material that will affect the phenotype in the next generation. This occurs during meiosis when the chromosomes segregate to the gametes. By chance, a proportion of gametes will have a balanced Robertsonian translocation or a normal chromosome complement. In others, the chromosome complement will be unbalanced because of a loss, or because of a duplication to a chromosome arm. Therefore, after fertilization, some zygotes will not be viable and this may manifest as recurrent miscarriages or infertility in carriers of Robertsonian translocations. The gain of additional chromosome 21q material because of this mechanism, is the cause of about 4 per cent of cases of Down syndrome; it occurs in children born to mothers with a Robertsonian translocation that affects chromosome 21.

Modern cytogenetic and molecular genetic techniques such as FISH, CGH, and WGS, have helped to identify the genetic causes of several previously unexplained syndromes. These *Contiguous Gene Syndromes* are referred to as submicroscopic because they are often undetectable by conventional karyotype analysis, using Giemsa staining and light microscopy. They are caused by deletions or, much less commonly, duplications of small chromosome regions. The commonest condition, affecting 1:4,000 live births, is 22q11.2 deletion syndrome, which had previously been recognized as *Di George syndrome*. The phenotype includes a combination of features; distinctive appearance, cleft palate, metabolic and immunological problems, and congenital heart disease. However, the clinical picture is hugely variable, and not uncommonly, making the diagnosis in an infant leads to recognition of an affected but asymptomatic parent. Accurate genetic diagnosis has led to considerable expansion of the phenotype of the condition, to include autoimmune disease, autism, and psychiatric disorders, notably schizophrenia. Manifestations are determined to some extent by the precise location of the microdeletion, which can be inherited or arise *de novo*.

The detection of the underlying 22q11 mutation using FISH is illustrated in Figure 4.8.

❯ which were introduced in Chapter 3.

Figure 4.8 DiGeorge syndrome—22q11 deletion—detected using FISH.
Wessex Reg. Genetics Centre/ Wellcome Collection CC-BY.

Human chromosomes have been stained with fluorescent probes. The probes bind
to specific sequences of DNA on chromosome 22. There has been a deletion in the
chromosome 22 indicated with an arrow. A control probe marks the telomeres of
both 22 homologues. A diagnostic probe can only been seen on one chromosome
22 homologue and has identified the hemizygous deletion at 22q11.

Key Points

- Chromosome abnormalities are a common cause of pregnancy loss and are
  present in approximately 1 per cent of newborn infants. Numerical and structural chromosomal mutations (including microdeletions) lead to a range of
  well-characterized phenotypes and are a common cause of learning disability. Down syndrome is the most common autosomal chromosomal syndrome.

Parent of Origin Effects: Imprinting and Uniparental Disomy

Angelman and Prader–Willi syndromes are separate disorders that are associated with the phenotypes described in Table 4.7. They are often considered
together because their underlying genetic causes involve genes that are closely
located on chromosome 15, and which are affected by genomic imprinting.
Imprinting results from epigenetic silencing of specific genes, usually by methylation, determined by the parent of origin. Many human gene loci are im-
printed, and in every case, correct gene dosage relies on inheritance of both
maternal and paternal alleles.

Angelman and Prader–Willi syndromes usually arise from deletion of the
chromosome region *15q11–13*, but the disease is determined by the originat-
ing chromosome. Angelman's syndrome affects around 1:12,000 children, and
is characterized by severe learning difficulties, severe epilepsy, absent speech,
inappropriate laughter and ataxia. Deletion of the *maternally-expressed* gene
UBE3A gene results in the condition in the majority of cases.

Table 4.7 Examples of microdeletion syndromes.

Microdeletion Location	Clinical Features
1q21.1	**TAR syndrome (T**hrombocytopenia and **A**bsent **R**adius). Thrombocytopenia (low platelets) usually improves with time. Many also have hypoplasia of the ulna. 50% have lactose intolerance.
1p36	**1p36 Deletion syndrome.** Growth failure, sensorineural hearing loss, progressive cardiomyopathy, hypothyroidism, seizures, severe intellectual disability.
5q35	**Soto syndrome.** Tall stature with macrocephaly, large hands and feet, hypotonia, clumsiness, intellectual disability.
7q11.23	**Williams syndrome.** Characterized by hypercalcaemia in infancy, often with failure to thrive, and characteristic 'elfin' faces and supravalvar aortic stenosis, or other cardiac anomalies
11p13	**WAGR syndrome.** Predisposition to Wilm's Tumour, Aniridia, Genito-urinary anomalies, intellectual disability.
Maternal 15q11–13	**Angelman syndrome.** Severe epilepsy, absent speech, hypotonia, feeding difficulties, ataxia, sleep disturbances, inappropriate laughter, severe intellectual disability (see text).
Paternal 15q11–13	**Prader–Willi syndrome.** Severe hypotonia and feeding difficulties at birth, voracious appetite and obesity in infancy, short stature, hypogonadism, intellectual disability (see text).
17p11.2	**Smith–Magenis syndrome.** Distinctive appearance, cleft palate, myopia, short stature, self-harming behaviour, intellectual disability.
22q11.2	**22q11.2 Deletion syndrome** (also known as Di George syndrome)**.** Cardiac anomalies, cleft palate, thymic hypoplasia, hypoparathyroidism, variable learning disabilities, schizophrenia, and other psychiatric disorders.
Xp21.2–p21.3	Duchenne muscular dystrophy, retinitis pigmentosa, adrenal insufficiency, intellectual disability, hypoglycaemia.

Children with Prader–Willi syndrome, which has a prevalence of 1:20,000, have a completely different phenotype with mild-to-moderate learning difficulties, severe hypotonia with poor feeding in infancy, but later severe hyperphagia and morbid obesity. In 70 per cent of cases, Prader–Willi syndrome results from a contiguous gene deletion affecting the genes *SNURF*, *SNRPN* and other genes on the *paternally derived* chromosome 15.

A small proportion of cases of Angelman and Prader–Willi syndromes result from a phenomenon known as uniparental disomy (UPD). In this situation, both copies of chromosome 15 are inherited from one parent, which has the same functional effect as a deletion.

4.4   Principles for Genetic Testing

The clinical utility of a valid genetic test, is the ability of that test to be useful in a particular clinical setting. The clinical setting may be as a predictive test for relatives of an affected case; or as a prenatal screening test; or a diagnostic test that confirms a particular diagnosis, or helps to resolve a differential diagnosis. There are many ways that an accurate genetic diagnosis could be useful in these settings:

❯ see whole genome analysis described in Chapter 3

- to assist the decision making about a medical or surgical treatment plan;
- to end a diagnostic odyssey and be of social or psychological value even in the absence of a specific treatment;
- to help with reproductive choices;
- to avoid harm; halting risky diagnostic procedures and interventions.

❯ see whole genome analysis described in Chapter 3.

Proper counselling of the family is needed, so they are aware of the possible ramifications of a particular result. When using broad tests such as CGH microarrays or WES and WGS, it is also important to consider the possibility of

Case Study 4.3
A complex genetic consultation

Caroline consulted a geneticist because her nephew, Oscar, had just been diagnosed with the X-linked condition, Duchenne Muscular Dystrophy (DMD). Caroline was concerned about her unborn child, her seven-year-old daughter Emma, and particularly her four-year-old son Harry, as she is aware of the risk of DMD in boys. Harry has speech delay and is somewhat clumsy.

Oscar's mother, Joanna, is well. It was unknown at that point whether she was a carrier for DMD, or whether Oscar's mutation arose *de novo*. If she was a carrier, she would most likely have inherited it from her mother.

Given the time constraint of Caroline's pregnancy, the geneticist opted to test Harry with a simple blood test, creatine kinase (CK), which is diagnostically elevated in DMD.

Unfortunately, the CK was very high confirming that Harry had DMD. This was subsequently confirmed by molecular genetic analysis of the dystrophin gene. This genetic test also confirmed by inference that Caroline and Joanna, and their mother, must be carriers.

Caroline's routine anomaly scan scheduled for twenty weeks was expedited and showed that she was carrying a girl (who therefore would not be affected). Caroline and John had detailed genetic counselling and they are not planning further children. They were concerned about the possibility of Emma being a carrier, as female carriers do exhibit progressive myopathy weakness in old age. However, as she will not have any health consequences in childhood, the parents were advised that Emma herself would have to decide whether to be tested, when she was of sufficient maturity to decide.

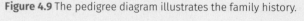

Figure 4.9 The pedigree diagram illustrates the family history.

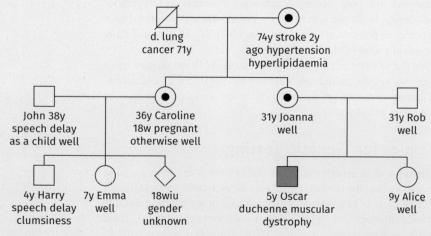

generating incidental findings that are unrelated to the reason for the test. Ideally, the consent process will include a discussion of whether the family wishes to be informed of such findings. Another consideration is the age of the patient. Professional genetics societies in Europe and North America recommend that genetic testing of children should be postponed until the child is old enough to make their own decisions about predictive testing, unless disease prevention or treatment opportunities would be missed by deferring the test. Look at the situation for Caroline and her daughter Emma illustrated in Case Study 4.3.

Prenatal screening for aneuploidy in the UK has been offered to women who are at increased risk of having a fetus affected by Down syndrome. This strategy detects approximately 60 per cent of the cases of Down syndrome. Of the ~10,000 women identified to be at higher risk each year, around 8,000 agree to amniocentesis, and approximately fifty of them will subsequently experience a miscarriage; which is a well-known complication of invasive prenatal sampling. However, in 2017, NIPT was introduced using a simple blood sample for the analysis of cell-free fetal DNA (cffDNA) to detect trisomy.

> See the Bigger Picture Panel 3.2 about NIPT in Chapter 3, which includes an interview with the medical sociologist, Professor Tom Shakespeare.

NIPT is more accurate than previous screening tests. False negatives (missed diagnoses) may occur (~0.3 per cent) because cffDNA comes from the placenta, and the fetal genotype may differ, or there may be inadequate fetal DNA obtained. However, it is anticipated that a smaller number of women will need to be offered amniocentesis (with the consequential risk of miscarriage). NIPT will also detect Patau syndrome, Edwards syndrome, and Turner syndrome. Commercial providers are already using this approach to offer NIPT for other genetic disorders, including 22q11 deletion syndrome.

Indications for Genetic Testing in Paediatric Medicine

Review the clinical reasons and typical scenarios for using genetic testing in Table 4.8. In addition to these scenarios, urgent testing is sometimes of the utmost importance, particularly for the newborn. The circumstances for these include the following.

- Severe lethal genetic abnormality, for instance suspected trisomy 13 or 18 in a child who would otherwise need life-saving surgery. In this situation, knowledge of the life-limiting diagnosis allows fully informed decision-making in the child's best interest.

- A child with a disorder of sex development, where the infant's sex cannot be determined clinically.

- A critically ill child with unexplained symptoms or disease. Approximately 5 per cent of infants admitted to neonatal intensive care will die. Sometimes, the cause is not evident. Rapid WES or WGS may yield an actionable diagnosis resulting in life-saving therapy, or at least yield a diagnosis allowing proper counselling of the family. Diagnostic yields, i.e. the proportion of tests that result in a definitive diagnosis, are high in this group (over 50 per cent in most studies). WES was first employed in 2011 to diagnose a child with an unsuspected immunodeficiency disorder, enabling a life-saving stem cell transplant to be performed. Subsequently, techniques have been refined, with some labs able to provide results in less than fifty hours. In many instances, the diagnosis is completely unanticipated, due to the rarity of the condition, or atypical presentations, emphasizing the merit of using genome and exome sequencing, rather than targeted tests.

> See *Bethany's diagnostic odyssey* in Chapter 3.

- In 2018, NHS England started a programme of WGS in the UK for children with severe undiagnosed conditions—including birth abnormalities, neurological symptoms including epilepsy, metabolic diseases or reduced growth.

Table 4.8 Indications for genetic testing.

Indication	Sign or Symptom	Examples of Genetic Conditions
Confirmation of a genetic disorder detected with pre-natal analysis	CVS, amniocentesis, and NIPT may identify chromosomal and other genetic disorders. It is usually appropriate to confirm the diagnosis after birth. Confirmation may take the form of genetic or biochemical tests, depending on the diagnosis under consideration.	Down syndrome
Prenatal ultrasound findings and abnormal intra-uterine growth	Some abnormal ultrasound findings possibly indicating genetic disease, e.g. short limbs, may not be obvious on the twenty-week fetal anomaly scan.	Achondroplasia
	Some genetic syndromes are associated with *in utero* growth restriction (IUGR).	Russell–Silver syndrome
	Some genetic syndromes are associated with a fetus that is large for its gestational age (LGA).	Beckwith–Wiedemann syndrome
Congenital anomalies	Distinctive physical features and morphological anomalies (*dysmorphology*) are associated with many genetic diseases and syndromes.	Edwards syndrome, Patau syndrome, and Down syndrome
Disorders in consanguineous families	First cousins will have approximately 12.5% of their DNA in common, and this may be higher if there are preceding consanguineous relationships.	AR disease such as the haemoglobinopathies
Neuromuscular diseases	Severe muscle weakness (*hypotonia*), abnormal gait, or seizures.	Muscular dystrophies and ataxia
Biochemical abnormalities	There are many inborn errors of metabolic processing which result in a range of abnormal biochemical signs from hypoglycaemia to failure to thrive. Only a small number are identified as a result of neonatal screening.	Congenital adrenal hypoplasia, cystic fibrosis, phenylketonuria
Neurocutaneous syndromes	Neurological signs such as seizures and learning difficulties, coupled with pathognomonic skin signs, such as café-au-lait patches.	Neurofibromatosis and tuberous sclerosis
Organ specific diseases	Any tissue or organ may be affected by genetic disease. The nature of the disease may point precisely to the diagnosis.	Osteogenesis imperfecta (history of low trauma fractures). Galactosemia (cataracts and liver dysfunction).
Abnormal post-natal growth & early onset obesity	Growth failure or excessive growth may point to a genetic disorder.	Turner syndrome Klinefelter syndrome Beckwith–Wiedemann syndrome Prader–Willi syndrome

Indication	Sign or Symptom	Examples of Genetic Conditions
Disorders of Sexual Development & Puberty	Many disorders of sexual development (DSD) manifest at birth with genital ambiguity, but others are not apparent until later, and may present with absent or delayed puberty.	Androgen insensitivity
Developmental Delay, Learning Disability & Autism	This group is one of the most challenging in terms of identifying genetic disease. Most affected children have no genetic diagnosis. This group was amongst the first to be investigated with WES, and diagnostic yields of 25% are reported.	See *Bethany's diagnostic odyssey* in Chapter 3.
Cancer	The most common symptom of Retinoblastoma is poor vision and a red or inflamed eye. The most common symptom of Wilms tumour is a swollen abdomen.	Retinoblastoma Wilms tumour

Chapter Summary

- The use of a pedigree diagram provides a standard, concise method for recording details of a family history. Completed diagrams are used to interpret patterns of inheritance for the phenotype of interest.
- Monogenic disorders show typical patterns of inheritance depending on whether they are caused by dominant or recessive mutations in X-linked, autosomal, or mitochondrial loci.
- The term *syndrome* is used when a group of clinical signs and symptoms occur together in a condition. Down syndrome is the most common autosomal chromosomal disorder; it is usually caused by trisomy 21 but in rare cases, an unbalanced structural abnormality is the underlying mutation. Numerical sex-chromosome abnormalities include Klinefelter syndrome in males, and Turner syndrome in females.
- Monogenic and chromosomal abnormalities lead to a large burden of disease and disability in childhood; including most cases of severe learning difficulty.
- Genetic analysis is used in prenatal screening; to confirm diagnoses in symptomatic children; and most recently to analyse whole genomes to identify mutations in critically ill infants to guide treatment decisions.

Discussion Questions

4.1 List three ways that a family history (pedigree) diagram can be helpful for the management of genetic disease.

4.2 Do you have brown eyes? Try representing yourself and your relatives in a three-generation family history (pedigree) diagram with respect to the trait of eye colour, or an alternative selected trait.

4.3 Do X-linked recessive diseases affect females? Explain your reasoning.

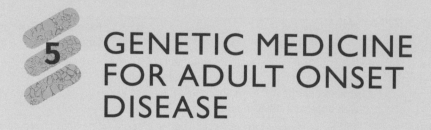

5 GENETIC MEDICINE FOR ADULT ONSET DISEASE

Learning Objectives

By the end of this chapter, you should be able to:

- discuss the concept of variable penetrance;
- explain the use of genetic testing for type 1 hereditary haemochromatosis;
- compare diseases with monogenic, polygenic, and multi-factorial causes;
- compare discontinuous and continuous traits;
- discuss the methods used to identify alleles with additive effects on complex disease phenotypes;
- explain what a polygenic risk score (PRS) is.

Genetic variants result in monogenic and common, **multifactorial** diseases that are diagnosed in adulthood. The underlying mutations may lead to a toxic accumulation of damaging gene products, or an absence of vital components of physiological pathways, over decades of life.

Huntington disease (HD), Type 1 Hereditary Haemochromatosis (HH), familial hypercholesterolaemia (FH), and family cancer syndromes are presented in this chapter, and summarized in Table 5.1, because they are instructive examples of monogenic disorders. Their causative mutations, and the associated pathology of each disease are well characterized. HD is a very rare disease, whereas HH and FH are often described as the most common genetic disorders in populations of European ancestry. Cancer is also a common condition of adulthood and it arises from a multistep accumulation of somatic mutations. However, for a small proportion of cancers, the disease is familial and shows an autosomal dominant inheritance pattern.

We discuss the frequency, origin, and nomenclature for the alleles that cause genetic disease in adulthood, along with the **penetrance** of the causative genotypes. Incomplete penetrance can arise if modifying variants or environmental factors have a role in the disease; these can suppress or enhance a phenotype.

The most common diseases of adulthood, such as coronary artery disease (CAD), cancer and dementia have a multifactorial cause. Their **genetic architecture** is usually complex, and the risk of symptomatic disease can be increased or decreased by lifestyle and other environmental influences. Most of the **heritability** of these common diseases can be explained by the additive and interactive effects of many genetic variants; which is **polygenic** inheritance. Some multifactorial diseases are associated with a significant disease burden in most populations. It has been proposed that predictive **polygenic risk scores** for these disorders will guide personalized and preventive medicine in the future.

5.1   Variable Penetrance

The term penetrance has been defined previously as the proportion of individuals with a disease-associated genotype who manifest the phenotype. The linked term, **expressivity**, is the degree to which the phenotype is expressed, or the extent of the manifestations in a given individual. In the genetic research literature, penetrance is increasingly used as an umbrella term for variations in all of the qualitative and quantitative clinical manifestations of a phenotype.

Many adult-onset monogenic diseases have variable ages of presentation and variable clinical manifestations. This may be due to differences between people and because the disease phenotype results from a complex set of genetic and environmental interactions. This conflicts with the notion that a particular mutation in a single gene is both essential **and sufficient** to cause the disease. However, many monogenic traits are modified by additional genetic loci.

In the study of monogenic diseases, the initial estimates of the lifetime penetrance of particular genotypes were made from studies of patients and their family members. However, as the use of genetic testing and DNA sequencing has increased for large control population cohorts, scientists have been surprised by the number of apparently unaffected individuals who have disease-associated genotypes.

Differences in the severity of a disease and its presentation may be explained by variability in the underlying mutations that cause monogenic disease; that is, some alleles or genotypes are more pathogenic than others. See Scientific Approach Panel 5.1 explaining a study of the pathogenicity of *BRCA1* mutations.

> these are also described in Table 5.1.

> The problems of data interpretation from genome sequencing were explored in Chapter 3.

Scientific Approach Panel 5.1
Classifying variants of *BRCA1* with the help of genome editing

Inherited germline mutations of the *BRCA1* gene may dramatically increase the risk of early onset breast and ovarian cancer. Because of this risk, more than 1 million women worldwide have had their *BRCA1* tumour suppressor genes analysed for variants that may be pathogenic. But there is a problem for risk preduction associated with newly characterized variants; thousands of different mutations have been identified in this large gene, and some mutations are classified as variants of unknown significance (VUS).

Patients may be alerted to VUS identified in their data but without an associated clinical risk prediction, the information may not be useful for their future healthcare. Laboratory and bioinformatics tools can improve risk-prediction. In 2018, a study by Findlay et al. was published describing a laboratory method that could be used to sub-classify variants according to pathogenicity. This method of sub-classification could help in the risk prediction of VUS.

The research team established a HAP1 human cell line that requires *BRCA1* expression for cell survival. They tested 4,000 different mutations that they engineered into the thirteen exons of the *BRCA1* gene of the cells' DNA, and by assaying cell survival, they were able to predict the pathogenicity of the variant. They compared their data about individual variants, with functional classifications for the same mutation from clinical databases. They found a very good correlation between their findings from the *in vitro* tissue culture model and the clinical classification of the mutations.

One really interesting feature of the study was the use of a gene editing system called **CRISPR** to create the mutations *in vitro*. CRISPR is an abbreviation of Clustered Regularly Interspaced Short Palindromic Repeats, which are part of a bacterial defence system, protecting them from foreign DNA. The term is also used for a genome editing technology that is based on the bacterial system. CRISPR editing is used widely in molecular genetic research laboratories to permanently modify genes in living cells and organisms and has been developed from a thorough understanding of the CRISPR mechanism of microbial defence.

CRISPR gene editing technology includes a short guide RNA sequence and a nuclease enzyme (e.g. Cas9). The nuclease introduces double-strand breaks into DNA, which will be repaired; specific sequence modifications can be made in conjunction with this approach, making it a useful genome-editing tool. The researchers investigating *BRCA1* mutations incorporated a plasmid, which they engineered to co-express the Cas9 enzyme and a guide RNA for the *BRCA1* gene, into the HAP1 cells.

In this study, the CRISPR technology was a powerful tool to investigate the pathogenicity of *BRCA1* mutations in an *in vitro* model. In the future, CRISPR technology may be also used for gene therapy *in vivo*, to correct mutations at precise locations in the human genome in order to treat genetic disease.

In 2020, clinical trials are under way to use CRISPR gene editing, in the hope of curing single gene disorders, including a form of congenital blindness, and sickle cell disease. The safety and benefits of a CRISPR based medicine to treat a degenerative retinal disease, Leber congenital amaurosis, are being tested in children and adults in the first CRISPR clinical trial in which gene editing takes place in the body. The CRISPR drug will be administered as a sub-retinal injection, with the aim of directly and permanently modifying the DNA of the photoreceptor cells.

Huntington Disease (HD) and Anticipation

❯ The class of the mutation and early onset HD are also discussed in Chapters 2 and 4.

The pathology of HD, which is a neurodegenerative disorder, is caused by an increase in the number of glutamine residues at the amino-terminus of the Huntingtin protein. The vast majority of cases of Huntington disease are diagnosed in adulthood—the average age of symptom onset is forty years. Signs and symptoms can include mood changes, small involuntary movements, poor coordination, and trouble learning new information or making decisions.

The underlying mutation is illustrated in Figure 5.1. It results in an increase in the number of CAG repeats in exon 1 of the coding DNA, and is referred to as a triplet repeat expansion. In the universal genetic code CAG specifies the amino acid glutamine, therefore the expanded CAG repeat is translated into an extended polyglutamine tract in the protein sequence.

❯ the code is illustrated in Figure 1.14

HTT alleles which result in a protein with forty or more glutamine residues, are associated with a toxic gain of function, and there is close to 100 per cent disease penetrance. We see a progressively earlier age of onset in the younger generations of some families affected by HD; this phenomenon of anticipation is because the triplet-repeat expansion is a dynamic mutation and it can expand during cell division, particularly in male meiotic divisions.

Type I Hereditary Haemochromatosis (HH) and Iron Overload

Type 1 HH is an autosomal recessive disorder caused by mutations in the *HFE* gene (see Case Study 5.1 about a family affected by HH). The disease alters iron homeostasis, through excessive absorption of dietary iron. Because there is no physiological mechanism for the excretion of excess iron, HH is characterized by iron overload and raised levels of the storage and transport molecules, ferritin and transferrin. HH is unusual among genetic diseases because it can be treated simply, to reduce the morbid disease consequences. Quantitative phlebotomy (the removal of blood) is illustrated in Figure 5.2, and is used to remove excess iron from the body's stores and so reduce damaging iron overload.

Table 5.1 Examples of monogenic diseases of adulthood.

Disease and Gene Locus	OMIM Entry	Mode of Inheritance	Class of Mutation	Prevalence of Disease or Pathogenic Mutations	Penetrance of Mutations
HD is caused by mutations to the *HTT* gene, its locus is on the short arm of chromosome 4	OMIM number #143100	Autosomal Dominant Inheritance Pattern shows *anticipation*.	Toxic gain of function mutation	Prevalence is approximately 1/10,000 but varies globally	High penetrance mutations with respect to morbidity and mortality. Penetrance is close to 100% for alleles with ≥ 40 CAG repeats
Type 1 HH is caused by mutations to the *HFE* gene, its locus is on the short arm of chromosome 6	OMIM Number #235200	Autosomal Recessive Inheritance Pattern	Loss of function mutations are Founder mutations	~ 1/250 have the at risk genotype in populations of northern European ancestry. Diagnosed HH is much less prevalent	Estimates of penetrance for disease manifestations vary from < 5% to > 20 % for pathogenic genotypes. Penetrance in p.C282Y homozygotes is greater than the penetrance in p.C282Y/p.H63D compound heterozygotes
FH is caused by mutations to *LDLR* gene on the short arm of chromosome 19	OMIM Number #143890	Autosomal Co-dominant	Loss of function mutations	1/250 have the at risk genotype in north American populations. Diagnosed FH is much less prevalent	Variable penetrance. Susceptibility affected by genetic and lifestyle modifiers
FAP is caused by mutations to the *APC* gene, its locus is on the long arm of chromosome 5	OMIM Number #175100	Autosomal Dominant Inheritance Pattern	Loss of function truncating mutations of the *APC* gene	Prevalence of FAP is approximately 2.3-3.2/100000 in the general population	Penetrance in mutation carriers is greater than 90%, but there is a wide range of clinical variability
Familial Breast and Ovarian Cancer Syndrome	OMIM Numbers #604370 #612555	Autosomal Dominant Inheritance Pattern	*BRCA1* *BRCA2* There is a great deal of heterogeneity in the position and type of pathogenic mutation to these loci between affected families. Most are truncating loss of function mutations	Prevalence estimates in the general population range from 1/200 to 1/800	Breast cancer risk by age 70 estimated to be ~ 70%, and the lifetime risk of ovarian cancer is lower. The penetrance of *BRCA1* mutations is higher than the penetrance of *BRCA2* mutations

HD: Huntington disease, HH: hereditary haemochromatosis, FH: Familial haemochromatosis, FAP: familial adenomatous polyposis. OMIM#: catalogue entry for Online Mendelian Inheritance in Man.

Figure 5.1 Huntington disease is caused by an expansion of a CAG (triplet-) repeat in the *HTT* gene.

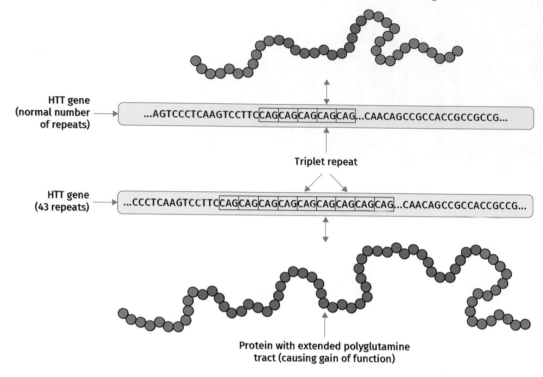

HTT gene
(normal number
of repeats) → ...AGTCCCTCAAGTCCTTCCAGCAGCAGCAGCAG...CAACAGCCGCCACCGCCGCCG...

Triplet repeat

HTT gene
(43 repeats) → ...CCCTCAAGTCCTTCCAGCAGCAGCAGCAGCAGCAGCAGCAG...CAACAGCCGCCACCGCCG...

**Protein with extended polyglutamine
tract (causing gain of function)**

Illustration based on original ideas courtesy of Health Education England's Genomics Education Programme.

Case Study 5.1
A family affected by hereditary haemochromatosis

Valerie Lundt is a thirty-seven-year-old woman who visited her general practitioner (GP) in Norfolk, East Anglia. She brought copies of genetic reports from family members to discuss. Each report recommended that she and other adult family members should be screened with a genetic test.

The reports relate to her older brothers, William and David. William is being treated for HH by regular quantitative phlebotomy and he has liver disease. Valerie's parents died in a car accident in 1998, they were forty-five and forty-seven years of age at the time. Valerie's GP

arranges for her to have a genetic test for mutations in the *HFE* gene. Table 5.2 lists the clinical reasons, results, and interpretation for the genetic tests completed for David, William, and Valerie.

Discussion Points

- Look at the results from the genetic reports and consider the genotypes of these three siblings.
- What assumptions can you make about the *HFE* genotypes of Valerie's mother and father?

Figure 5.2 Signs and symptoms and treatment of hereditary haemochromatosis. (a) The clinical manifestations of HH include biochemical evidence of iron overload and excessive iron storage in the liver, skin, heart, joints and the testes. This can cause abdominal pain, cirrhosis and liver cancer, arthritis, cardiomyopathy, and hypogonadism. Clinical manifestations are more common in men than women. (b) HH can be treated by phlebotomy, to remove excess iron from the body.

(a)

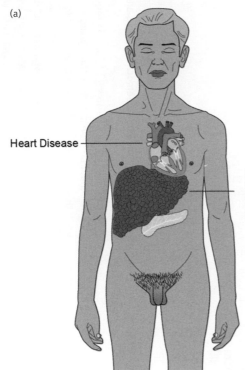

Heart Disease

Hepatomegaly
Elevated Liver Enzymes
Cirrhosis
Hepatocellular carcinoma

Laboratory Test Results

- Raised serum iron and transferrin saturation
- Raised serum ferritin
- Liver biochemistry abnormalities
- Liver biopsy shows increased iron deposition
- Endocrine abnormalities
- Mutations of *HFE* gene

(b)

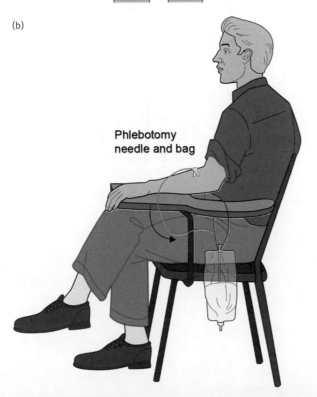

Phlebotomy
needle and bag

Table 5.2 A summary of data from the genetics laboratory reports.

Name and date of birth (d.o.b.)	Clinical Details	Result from Genetic Report	Interpretation & Advice on the Report
William Lundt (d.o.b. 28/02/73)	Elevated ferritin levels & abnormal liver function tests	**HFE p.C282Y homozygous** DNA was extracted and tested using a PCR and restriction digest method that detects the two commonest mutations of the *HFE* gene: p.His63Asp (H63D) and p.Cys282Tyr (C282Y) (reference sequence NM_000410.3)	The patient has two copies of the C282Y mutation of the *HFE* gene. The H63D mutation is not present **This genotype is strongly associated with type 1 haemochromatosis.** The patient should have a fasting transferrin saturation and ferritin tests. If currently normal, these should be repeated annually Many patients with this genotype will require regular phlebotomy to prevent iron overload. A specialist referral is suggested This genotype is found in 90% of patients with haemochromatosis in the UK. However, in some individuals this genotype does not cause clinical symptoms, hence other causes of any clinical symptoms should also be considered Relatives of the patient, particularly siblings, are also at risk of haemochromatosis. The patient should be advised that *HFE* testing is available for relatives. Testing of children under 16 is not recommended
David Lundt (d.o.b. 27/03/75)	Family history of HH	**HFE p.C282Y heterozygous** DNA was extracted and tested using a PCR and restriction digest method that detects the two commonest mutations of the *HFE* gene: p.His63Asp (H63D) and p.Cys282Tyr (C282Y) (reference sequence NM_000410.3)	David carries a single p.C282Y mutation. He is not at greater risk of iron overload than the general population, but is a carrier so screening of adult family members might be considered
Valerie Lundt (d.o.b 02/04/81)	Family history of HH	**HFE p.C282Y/p.H63D compound heterozygous** DNA was extracted and tested using a PCR and restriction digest method that detects the two commonest mutations of the *HFE* gene: p.His63Asp (H63D) and p.Cys282Tyr (C282Y) (reference sequence NM_000410.3)	The patient has one copy of the C282Y mutation and one copy of the H63D mutation of the *HFE* gene **This genotype is associated with type 1 haemochromatosis and clinically significant iron overload** The patient should have a fasting transferrin saturation and ferritin tests. If currently normal, these should be repeated every three years Some patients with this genotype will require regular phlebotomy to maintain a normal ferritin level. A specialist referral should be considered This genotype is found in about 5% of patients with haemochromatosis in the UK. This genotype is found in about 2% of the East Anglian population. In most individuals this genotype does not cause clinical symptoms. Hence, other possible causes of any clinical symptoms should also be considered Relatives of the patient, particularly siblings, may have a genotype associated with risk of iron overload. The patient should be advised that *HFE* testing is available for relatives. Testing of children under 16 is not recommended

Two missense SNVs of the *HFE* gene are found in patients with the most common type of HH. The majority of patients are homozygous for a mutation that leads to a change at amino acid 282 of the HFE protein. A small number of patients are compound heterozygotes; they carry the variant that causes the 282 amino acid change and a variant on their other *HFE* allele, which alters amino acid 63 of the protein. A few other *HFE* SNPs and examples of private *HFE* mutations have been associated with rare cases and families affected by HH. Both variants are founder mutations. Both mutations have the same common variants in the DNA that flanks the *HFE* gene: this is evidence that all individuals with one of these mutations share a common single ancestor.

❯ The Founder effect is explained in Chapter 2.

The pathogenic mutant genotypes have variable expressivity and low penetrance with respect to some disease manifestations caused by iron overload. These disease manifestations are associated with high morbidity, and include liver cirrhosis and liver cancer. One of the pathogenic genotypes (p.C282Y homozygosity) has a higher penetrance with respect to morbidity than the compound heterozygous genotype. In the Scientific Approach Panel 5.2 there is a discussion about age-related penetrance that has implications for managing HH to prevent life-threatening disease manifestations.

Familial Hypercholesterolaemia and Cascade Family Testing

Some cases of coronary artery disease (CAD) are caused by the monogenic trait FH. In the 1980s one genetic cause of FH was identified which was the inheritance of loss-of-function mutations in the gene that encodes the receptor for low-density lipoprotein (*LDLR*). When this receptor is impaired, it affects the uptake of cholesterol by the liver cells, and leads to raised levels of cholesterol in the circulation (hypercholesterolaemia). Mutations at other genetic loci also cause FH; disorders with the same phenotype arising from mutations at different loci are referred to as genocopies.

Figure 5.3 Founder, missense mutations in the *HFE* gene on the short arm of chromosome 6 were identified in 1996.

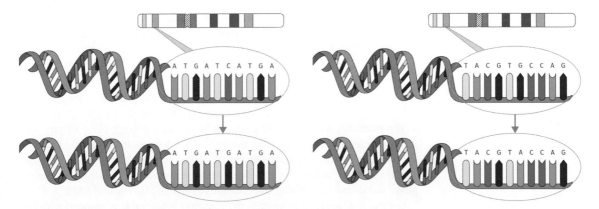

The p.H63D mutation results from a cytosine to guanine transition at nucleotide 187 of the DNA sequence of the *HFE* gene.

The p.C282Y mutation results from a transition from guanine to adenine at nucleotide 845 of the DNA sequence of the *HFE* gene. For the p.H63D mutation, there is a cytosine to guanine transition at nucleotide 187.

Scientific Approach Panel 5.2
UK Biobank and a cohort study of HH and disease manifestations

UK Biobank was set up in 2006, to improve the diagnosis, treatment, and prevention of many common illnesses of older age, including cancer, heart disease, and dementia.

It is a large project that will follow up the health of its participants over many years. By 2010, there were 500,000 participants aged between forty and sixty-nine. These volunteers have undergone tests and provided detailed information about themselves, including their family history. They have also provided blood and other samples for banking. Each participant agreed to the ongoing monitoring of their health records. The sample-banking and detailed data collection means that scientists can study the genetic and environmental causes of ill health.

One UK Biobank study by Pilling et al. in 2019 examined the frequency of disease diagnoses that are associated with the common underlying genotypes for HH.

We know that only a minority of individuals with the at-risk genotypes are diagnosed with haemochromatosis: is this a failure of HH diagnosis or are the *HFE* genotypes often non-penetrant? This question is important because HH is easily treatable, as illustrated in Figure 5.2.

Some of the questions addressed by the authors of the Biobank study consider this issue by asking;

- What disease manifestations are associated with HFE mutations?
- How many people with the at-risk genotypes get these manifestions, and when?

They found that for men with the p.C282Y homozygous genotype, liver disease, osteoporosis, arthritis, pneumonia, and diabetes were significantly more common at baseline. In both men and women, these disease manifestations occurred more commonly in mutant homozygotes during the follow-up period. They also concluded that an excess of these diseases is more common with advancing age.

At the end of the study, 75 per cent of the 2,980 participants with the p.C282Y homozygous genotype had not been diagnosed with HH. This could be interpreted as non-penetrance for the genotype, however, some had a diagnosis of an associated disease manifestation.

The UK Biobank participants are a population sample and so will include individuals with and without *HFE* mutations, and those with and without disease manifestations. A cohort study like this is a good design because it reduces some biases that can occur with a pre-selected group of diagnosed patients. The Biobank cohort cannot completely eliminate all bias, for example some of the p.C282Y homozygotes had already been diagnosed with HH when they joined the study, and individuals might have been motivated to participate because of their diagnosis.

This study confirms the known disease associations with *HFE* p.C282Y homozygosity and the relatively low penetrance of the mutations in women. This study design illustrates the difficulty of gathering data on a disease with a late onset. In a cohort study, only very long follow-up can avoid the pitfalls of recruiting a young population where disease is not apparent by the end of the study, or recruiting an older population where some at-risk individuals have already died.

The question of whether screening for *HFE* mutations would be beneficial remains open: some lives would be saved, but many people would receive expensive, burdensome, and unnecessary treatment. The balance is not yet clear.

The morbidity associated with FH can be reduced through early dietary and medical interventions, including the use of cholesterol-lowering medications such as statins. Cascade family testing is therefore used for the effective management of FH, and for other monogenic diseases which have a pre-symptomatic phase and disease-modifying interventions available (e.g. HH and FAP).

Genetic tests are used to identify the causative mutation in a proband with FH. This is followed by cascade family testing to identify other individuals who may be at risk of the disease before symptoms show. FH usually shows a dominant inheritance pattern, so first-degree relatives have a 50 per cent risk of carrying the causative mutation. Therefore, cascade testing targets the first-degree relatives of the affected individuals. If a relative has the same mutation as the proband, they become the proband for the next round of cascade screening. The results of the cascade screening can inform decisions about the use of statins and other treatments in patients with pre-symptomatic FH.

Family Cancer Syndromes and Tumour Suppressor Genes

Cancer is a common disease and caused by the multi-step accumulation of a critical number of mutations over the life course. Most changes that drive carcinogenesis are somatic mutations that affect two classes of genes in particular, the oncogenes and tumour suppressor genes (TSGs).

A small percentage of all cancers cluster in families and show a monogenic inheritance pattern, often with incomplete penetrance. In Table 5.1, familial forms of colorectal and breast cancer are presented as examples. A germline mutation in a TSG is the underlying cause of the very high cancer risk in these families.

The products of TSGs often regulate passage through the cell cycle and/or facilitate DNA repair. Physiologically, the TSG proteins may also regulate the balance between cell division and cell death (apoptosis). Loss of function somatic mutations (such as deletions or truncating mutations) of TSGs are commonly found in all types of sporadic and familial cancer. The impact of TSG mutations is recessive at the cellular level, so malignant phenotypes usually only occur if both alleles are mutated. In families with familial adenomatous polyposis or breast and ovarian cancer syndrome, affected individuals have inherited a critical first step in the process of carcinogenesis, which is a germline mutation in one TSG allele. But to observe the associated phenotype, somatic mutations or epigenetic changes have to occur to knock out the function of the other TSG allele.

> ❯ See Chapter 2 for a discussion of driver somatic mutations and cancer development; and Chapter 6 for a discussion of the use of personalized medicine in cancer.

Key Points

- Individuals who carry germline mutations to TSGs such as *APC* or *BRCA1* do not *all* develop cancer; they are simply at a much greater risk of developing the disease than individuals without these inherited mutations.

There are a number of signs that an individual, or members of a family, might have an inherited predisposition to cancer, including:

- several family members have the disease;
- cancer is diagnosed at a younger age than usual (e.g. below the age of 50);
- multifocal cancer, e.g. bilateral breast cancer.

The diagnosis and management of families affected by inherited cancer syndromes comprises a major part of the workload of a clinical genetics service. Interventions include surveillance for early signs and symptoms of disease; and treatment, including prophylactic medical and surgical interventions for pre-symptomatic disease.

5.2   Multifactorial Inheritance and the Liability Threshold Model

The inheritance of multifactorial traits results from the additive contributions of many genes (polygenic), or several genes (oligogenic) and their interaction with environmental factors. They do recur in families, but not in the pattern typical of monogenic disorders. These traits include:

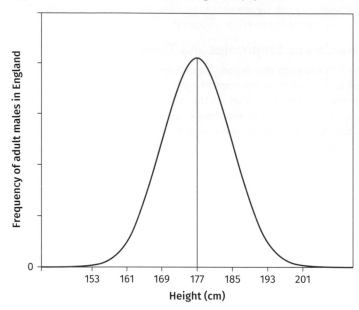

Figure 5.4 The normal distribution of height in a population.

- normal characteristics such as height and general intelligence;
- physiological factors such as blood pressure;
- diseases such as schizophrenia, type 2 diabetes mellitus (T2DM), arthritis, and coronary artery disease (CAD).

Multifactorial phenotypes can be subdivided into discontinuous and continuous traits. Discontinuous traits occur in discrete categories; being present or absent. The diagnosis of a disease is a categorical trait, as is an observation of a specific hair colour. In contrast to this, continuous traits are on a quantitative continuum; the differences between individuals differ by small degrees and show a normal distribution. The distribution of height in a population, illustrated in Figure 5.4, reflects the particular contribution of many genetic variants at different loci that exert an additive effect.

Whereas monogenic diseases have a predictable pattern of disease recurrence in families, even allowing for variable penetrance, the recurrence pattern is less predictable for polygenic and oligogenic traits. However, observations about family clustering and genetic risk for these more complex traits include:

- a higher recurrence rate in the relatives of the most severely affected cases (for example, those with a younger age of onset, and multifocal disease);
- the recurrence risk for first-degree relatives of an affected individual is roughly equal to the square root of the population incidence for the condition;
- the recurrence risk falls away steeply for second- and third-degree relatives in polygenic traits.

Heritability

❯ Genome-Wide Association Studies (GWAS) are introduced in Chapter 2.

Recent GWAS of height, in a cohort of 700,000 individuals, showed that about 500 genetic loci contributed to the heritability of height; heritability, being the proportion of phenotypic variance that is accounted for by genetic effects. Heritability is a population-specific measurement because variability between groups may differ by ethnicity and environmental influence. Non-genetic factors such as diet also contribute to the variance observed for multifactorial phenotypes such as height. The many loci that contribute to a continuous trait are known as quantitative trait loci, which is often abbreviated to QTL in research papers.

The heritability estimates for a number of multifactorial traits are shown in Table 5.3.

Heritability estimates for diseases are derived from an analysis of the recurrence risk within families, the aim being to apportion the effects of genetics and the effects of the environment and chance. Initial observations of the clustering of a phenotype may be followed by specific comparisons of the disease risk for first, second, and third-degree relatives. Twin studies represent the ultimate family study of heritability, because there is better control for the shared environments for the family members. In these studies, the phenotype concordance rates are compared for pairs of monozygotic and dizygotic twins; the twins are concordant for a phenotype if they are both affected. For multifactorial conditions, the concordance rates for monozygotic twins (who are almost genetically identical) are higher than the concordance rates for dizygotic twins (who only share ~ 50 per cent of their genes), but are less than 100 per cent because of environmental differences. If inherited genetic differences are not relevant to a trait, the concordance rates for monozygotic twins would be no different from the concordance rates for dizygotic twins.

Studies of the heritability of psychological traits have been carried out in large longitudinal follow-up studies of twins. Data shows that the heritability of these traits, from educational attainment to the development of schizophrenia or major depression, is approximately 50 per cent. This suggests that additive genetic variants explain 50 per cent of the variance between people for the psychological traits and psychiatric disorders studied.

Very large cohorts of patients have been studied in GWAS, with the aim of understanding the loci that contribute to the heritability of adult onset diseases. To date only a small proportion of the underlying additive genetic variants have been identified for most multifactorial traits. But with the analysis of *big data* from cohorts of hundreds of thousands of individuals, an understanding of the genetic architecture of these complex traits is growing.

Table 5.3 The heritability of common multifactorial diseases of adulthood from studies of UK and US populations.

Disease	Heritability Estimates
CAD	50%
T2DM	70%
Osteoarthritis	39% to 65%*
Late onset Alzheimer's Disease (AD)	50%
Schizophrenia	50%

Heritability is a statistical measure of the phenotypic variance within a population that is caused by genetic factors. CAD: coronary artery disease; T2DM: Type 2 Diabetes Mellitus. *Estimates for arthritis vary according to the site of the disease.

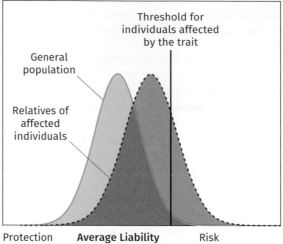

Figure 5.5 The impact of the liability threshold is compared for a family affected by a quantitative polygenic trait and for the general population.

The Liability Threshold Model

It is worth thinking about how categorical disease states, such as a diagnosis of diabetes or heart disease, can have an underlying oligogenic or polygenic genetic influence. Their cause has been explained by the Liability Threshold Model; which proposes that all additive factors (both polygenic and environmental) are considered as a liability. The disease manifestations occur when a certain threshold-of-liability is exceeded in an individual.

In Figure 5.5 the liability threshold is compared for an affected family and for the general population.

Data from GWAS of complex, multifactorial diseases have supported this model of liability because variants at tens or even hundreds of different loci are often associated with the diseases.

5.3   Complex Traits and Genetic Medicine

It is predicted that the application of genetics to medicine will have a much bigger impact on the management of multifactorial diseases than it already has on rare, monogenic, and chromosomal diseases. This is because the diseases are so common that any new genetic biomarkers or therapeutic pathways identified could lead to significant reductions in morbidity and mortality at a population level.

The remainder of this chapter will focus on the genetic architecture of common diseases of adulthood. Diseases may be largely monogenic traits that are modified by additional loci as described above or complex multifactorial traits, and many disease classifications span both. Understanding the number and effect sizes of the underlying mutations for a trait can result in the identification of new therapeutic pathways and models of predictive testing.

Late Onset AD and *APOE*

AD is the leading cause of dementia. Its prevalence in the population rises steeply with age; affecting between 10 and 15 per cent of the population by the age of eighty. More than forty GWAS have reproducibly identified variants in tens of loci with small or moderate effect sizes. However, the most significant risk factor in all populations are particular polymorphisms of the *APOE* gene. At least one high-risk allele, *APOE* e4, is found in more than 40 per cent of patients with late onset AD, and the lifetime risk of AD for individuals who are homozygous for the e4 variant is 80 per cent. This is a significant risk factor but it does not provide a viable genetic test for the complex trait to guide clinical management because most patients do not have this variant and not all people who carry the variant will develop the disease. However, there are commercial services for this and other common genetic risk factors that are offered as direct-to-consumer genetic tests, that is, without the intervention of a clinician and formal genetic counselling.

The identification of the *APOE* variants and other genetic risk factors has led to a greater understanding of the biological pathways altered in AD. These include lipid metabolism, inflammation, and other immune responses.

5.4 Coronary Artery Disease (CAD)

CAD is an important target for genetic medicine, because this complex phenotype is the leading cause of death worldwide.

Pathologically, CAD is the progressive build-up of fatty deposits in blood vessels, which leads to inflammatory responses, and narrowing of the arteries that supply the heart (this intermediate phenotype is called atherosclerosis). If CAD results in an obstruction to blood flow a myocardial infarction may occur which can result in cell death, damage to the heart muscle; and even death. Like most complex diseases that present in adulthood, CAD results from an interplay of lifestyle and genetic factors. The heritability of fatal and early-onset CAD is estimated to be approximately 50 per cent.

A clinically important association between elevated levels of plasma cholesterol with CAD is well established. Therapies such as statins are used to target the hypercholesterolaemia, including FH discussed earlier in this chapter, 'Familial Hypercholesterolaemia and Cascade Family Testing', and to prevent CAD and early death.

> including FH discussed earlier in this chapter.

Look at Figure 5.6, which illustrates the complexity of the metabolic pathways that statins affect. Mutations in several loci that encode the enzymes and receptors (e.g. the LDL receptor) within this pathway have been associated with increased CAD risk.

Important genes and pathways have certainly been identified by studying the DNA and phenotypes of families who had extreme manifestations of disease. However, most of our understanding of the genetic architecture of CAD has resulted from very large studies of patient populations to identify common and rare, additive risk factors.

 Key Points

- Although monogenic conditions such as FH result in CAD, most of its heritability is explained by polygenic factors.

Understanding the genetics of CAD and identifying targets for novel therapies

Genetic association studies of CAD have reproducibly identified common and rare variants in more than sixty distinct genetic loci. GWAS have been used to systematically compare the frequency of common variants in CAD cohorts and

Figure 5.6 Gene products that influence the effect of statins on hepatic cholesterol metabolism and plasma lipoprotein transport.

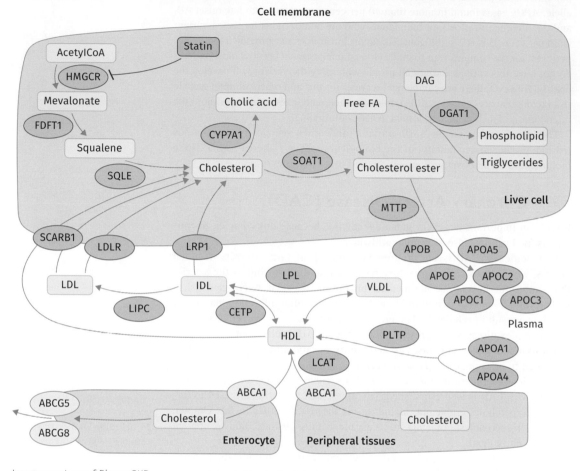

Image courtesy of PharmGKB.

disease-free control cohorts. Much of the heritability for CAD can be explained by common variants (with an allele frequency of > 5 per cent) that are each associated with a very small increased risk.

Interestingly, many of the variants lie in non-coding, regulatory regions of the genome, and therefore CAD risk factors often have a role in altering expression of genes at other loci. One of the first reproducible GWAS findings was the identification of variants of the *ANRIL* locus, which is found on the short arm of chromosome 9 (9p21). The non-coding *ANRIL* RNA alters the activity of two genes (*CDKN2A* and *CDKN2B*) that encode modulators of inflammatory signalling. This direct modulation of gene expression at one locus by the transcript of a different gene is an example of gene-gene interaction called epistasis. Interactions between genes can mean that the genotype from one gene locus can conceal, or enhance, the phenotype that arises from the genotype from a different gene locus. Epistatic interaction is observed when the gene products are part of the same metabolic pathway or transcription factor network. When gene products exert their phenotypic effects via distinct pathways the quantitative effects of mutations may be purely additive; however, most genes show some evidence of epistasis.

Understanding the links between genetic associations and disease mechanisms is important for demonstrating causality, and to identify potential treatment

❯ Non-coding genome elements are introduced in Chapter 1.

> ### 💡 Key Points
>
> - Polygenic inheritance and epistatic interactions mean that it is a challenge to isolate the impact of an individual gene on a particular complex phenotype. However, large GWAS studies have reproducibly identified loci that are associated with common diseases, such as CAD.

pathways. Data from GWAS have revealed that rare and common risk-modulating variants for CAD often affect loci that were already being targeted with cholesterol or hypertension-lowering therapies. These are reassuring findings that validate the GWAS approach. Perhaps most importantly, new therapeutic targets have been identified too; for example mutations in the *SORT1* gene have been identified as CAD risk factors. The *SORT1* gene product, sortilin, affects apolipoprotein B (APOB) secretion and LDL metabolism (see Figure 5.6 for the role of APOB in lipid metabolism; this protein is one component of LDL). Another important gene is *PCSK9*, because its product binds to the LDL receptor leading to its breakdown. Gain-of-function mutations in this gene cause FH because the LDL receptors can no longer remove cholesterol from the blood. Monoclonal antibodies directed against the PCSK9 protein and RNA inhibitors have been used in promising clinical trials. Genomic research is therefore identifying causal links for CAD-associated genetic variants and is driving the development and clinical trial of novel drugs.

Figure 5.7 An illustration of how genomic medicine can contribute to healthcare for cardiology patients. Genetic biomarkers are used in cascade family testing; rational drug design; pharmacogenetics, and assessing disease risk for patients with monogenic and chronic multifactorial diseases, including CAD.

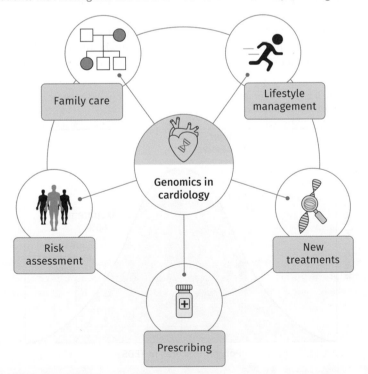

Illustration based on original ideas courtesy of Health Education England's Genomics Education Programme.

See Figure 5.7 for an illustration of the overall contribution that genomic medicine is making to CAD patients and others with complex, multifactorial diseases.

5.5   Will Polygenic Risk Scores (PRS) be Useful Clinically?

GWAS findings could have another clinical application, which is the generation of a predictive score for an individual's risk of developing CAD and other multifactorial diseases such as dementia, schizophrenia, and breast cancer; and non-disease traits such as height and educational attainment.

GWAS data coupled with data from large genetic epidemiological studies, like UK Biobank, are revealing the individual and additive impact of thousands or even millions of genetic variants on common disease phenotypes. Using the information from all of the GWAS genetic data points provides probabilistic information that is becoming known as a polygenic risk score or PRS. These predictive scores could be used to guide treatment and screening strategies in the future.

A PRS could be applied in the same way as existing predictive tests for monogenic disorders. For CAD, individuals with a high PRS have been shown to have a higher disease risk than individuals with a *LDLR* monogenic mutation. Breast cancer demonstrates a similar balance. Although *BRCA1* and *BRCA2* mutations can lead to a greatly increased risk of breast cancer in some families, most of the heritability of breast cancer comes from additive polygenic factors. It is proposed that PRS could improve the screening regimes for breast cancer in the general population. Women in the UK and the US join screening programmes, using mammography, at about fifty years of age to detect pre-symptomatic breast cancer. But some women at increased disease risk could be identified from their PRS, and might benefit from earlier screening, and the converse may be true for individuals with very low risk scores.

The psychologist and behavioural geneticist, Robert Plomin, recently published his own PRS profile. It was derived using population data collected as part of a large cohort study of twins for psychological traits, called the TEDS

Figure 5.8 Illustration of a psychological profile of polygenic risk scores for one individual.

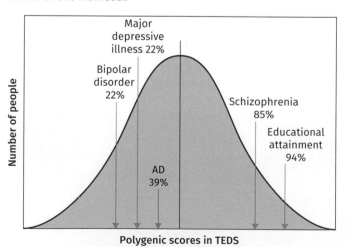

Image courtesy of Robert Plomin.

study. Figure 5.8 illustrates his educational attainment and schizophrenia scores at the higher end of the normal distribution, and his PRS scores for bipolar disorder, depression and AD that are lower than average.

One limitation for using PRS to plan interventions such as screening programmes or lifestyle modification is that the scores currently only explain a proportion of the heritability predicted for the traits. There is also a philosophical problem for their application because there is no clear causal pathway for most of the PRS variants associated with the disease traits. Ongoing research with larger cohorts may narrow the remaining gaps in knowledge and understanding.

Chapter Summary

- The diseases of adulthood have a varied genetic architecture. There are monogenic traits associated with a rare single high penetrance variant; monogenic traits that are modified by additional loci; and oligogenic or polygenic inheritance patterns, associated with many common variants, most with small individual effects.
- Modifying environmental factors affect the penetrance of the genotypes that cause rare monogenic disease and common multifactorial disease.
- Founder mutations in the *HFE* gene, that are common in individuals with European ancestry, cause the majority of cases of type 1 HH (OMIM entry #235200).
- The genetic variance observed for common multifactorial traits such as CAD can be explained by combinations of rare variants (with major effects) and common variants (with individually small effects).
- Understanding the genetic architecture of common multifactorial diseases is leading to the development of new diagnostic and treatment strategies. These may include the use of PRS for personalized medicine to guide treatment and screening.
- Genetic medicine will have a bigger impact on the management of multifactorial diseases than monogenic diseases. This is because the diseases are so common that any new genetic biomarkers or therapeutic pathways identified could lead to significant reductions in morbidity and mortality at a population level.

Further Reading

Review:

Claussnitzer, M., Cho, J. H., Collins, R., Cox, N. J., Dermitzakis, E. T., et al. (2020). A brief history of human disease genetics. Nature, 577, 179–89. https://www.nature.com/articles/s41586-019-1879-7

Discussion Questions

5.1 Review the case study about the family affected by HH. Draw a pedigree diagram to illustrate the family history described. What advice might Valerie's GP offer about the benefits and problems of genetic testing?

5.2 What factors could affect the penetrance of a mutation or genotype?

5.3 *All* diseases are multifactorial; discuss.

5.4 If tests for polygenic risk scores were available from your healthcare provider, would you request one? Discuss your reasoning.

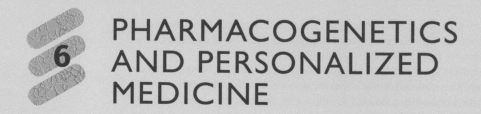

6 PHARMACOGENETICS AND PERSONALIZED MEDICINE

Learning Objectives

By the end of this chapter, you should be able to:

- define pharmacodynamics and pharmacokinetics.;
- discuss adverse events and the ethical principle 'to do no harm';
- explain actionable mutations in the development of cancer and companion diagnostics;
- define **pharmacogenomics**, and discuss the benefits and challenges of treatment stratification and personalized medicine.

Pharmacogenetics is an emerging branch of medical science. It is being used to improve the effectiveness of medicines, and to minimize their harmful side effects, the latter of which we refer to as adverse drug reactions (ADRs) throughout this chapter.

Panels of pharmacogenetic **biomarkers** are being used clinically to predict pharmacological response and to plan treatment regimes. These biomarkers can be for the analysis of both germline and somatic genetic variation.

We know that a 'one-size-fits-all' dose is not appropriate for many commonly prescribed drugs, because genetic variation affects how rapidly a drug is activated, or cleared, from our bodies, as well as the amount needed to be effective. Pharmacologists study both the action of drugs on target cells and tissues (**pharmacodynamics**) and the response of the body to the drug (**pharmacokinetics**). Genetic factors are important, because variations in proteins and protein pathways influence pharmacodynamics and pharmacokinetics. Furthermore, particular genetic variants are associated with susceptibility to severe hypersensitivity and very rare ADRs.

Where medical treatment damages health, it violates the key ethical principle of non-maleficence, and the oath that many doctors take 'to do no harm'. It has become a priority to understand ADRs at the molecular level, so that the risk of harm can be avoided.

6.1   The Historical Perspective

One pharmacogenetic trait that is linked to diet is called *favism*, and it has been documented for centuries. Favism is caused by an inborn error of metabolism, known as glucose-6-phosphate dehydrogenase (G6PD) enzyme deficiency, which can lead to acute *haemolytic anaemia* with exposure to certain drugs or dietary factors, including fava beans.

It is claimed that the ancient Greek philosopher, Pythagoras, noted this toxicity (or ADR) in some people, and warned against the consumption of the offending beans. The trait is particularly common in Mediterranean populations, because there is a high prevalence of G6PD deficiency and fava beans are widely consumed.

The underlying mutations to the gene *G6PD* results in a deficiency of the pentose phosphate pathway. This metabolic pathway produces sugars for nucleic acids, and NADPH, which is an important molecule for protecting cells from reactive oxygen species and cellular damage. A shortage of NADPH renders red blood cells, which have no mitochondria, particularly sensitive to oxidative stress, and this leads to their destruction and *haemolytic anaemia*. The acute anaemia can be induced by organic compounds found in both dietary components such as fava beans and in medicines, such as the anti-malarial treatment, primaquine.

G6PD is a gene on the X-chromosome. The G6PD-deficiency trait is referred to as a monogenic X-linked disorder.

> which is an inheritance pattern explored in Chapter 4.

Other enzyme deficiencies that cause drug toxicity can also be tracked in families as monogenic traits. For example, butyrylcholinesterase deficiency is an autosomal recessive condition. It leads to ADRs from the muscle relaxant suxamethonium chloride, which is used during general anaesthesia. Susceptible individuals take much longer than usual to clear choline ester drugs from the body because they lack a functional copy of the *BCHE* gene, and they may not be able to move or breathe without ventilation for hours after surgery. As the condition is rare, with approximately 1/5,000 people affected, biomarkers for the underlying mutations or for the enzyme deficiency are not routinely used before surgery. However, because of this and some other inherited traits, anaesthetists do ask new patients about their family history of general anaesthesia and ADRs.

6.2   Pharmacodynamics and Genetics

The term pharmacodynamics describes the biological effect of the drug on its target, which may include the physical binding of active metabolites and pro-drugs to one or more proteins. These proteins may be receptors, ion channels, enzymes and transporters and some examples are illustrated in Figure 6.1. A drug may inhibit a protein from binding to its normal ligand (the drug is therefore described as an **antagonist**), or the drug may activate a pathway (the drug is therefore described as an *agonist*), see Figure 6.1 (a) for an illustration. The pharmacodynamic effect of the drug is influenced by genetics because the proteins that are the drug targets within cells and tissues vary between individuals.

  Key Points

- The term pharmacodynamics describes the interaction between a drug and its molecular target or *what the drug does to the body.*

Pharmacogenetic biomarker test results can predict whether a drug will be beneficial for a patient; this is referred to as **efficacy**. In studies of biomarkers,

Figure 6.1 An illustration of pharmacodynamic and pharmacokinetic principles. (a) Pharmacodynamics. Examples of interactions between drug types and target proteins. (b) Pharmacokinetics. The absorption, distribution, metabolism and excretion (ADME) of an oral drug.

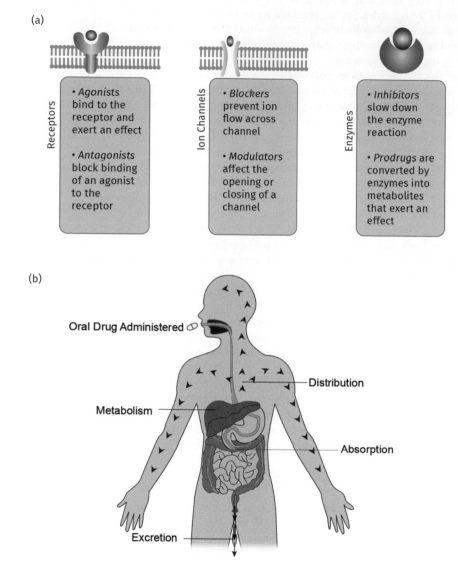

Figure 6.1 (a) was developed with guidance from Professor Yoon Loke, Professor of Clinical Pharmacology at Norwich Medical School.

efficacy is measured by enhanced survival or through the relief of the signs and symptoms of the disease, as compared to no drug or an alternative drug. See Scientific Approach Panel 6.1 to consider the signs and symptoms of cystic fibrosis that were monitored in the trials of ivacaftor.

Biomarkers can also be used to predict the dose of a drug required for an individual patient. A clinically important example of this aim is for the oral anticoagulant, warfarin, as described in Case Study 6.1. This commonly prescribed drug interferes with (antagonizes) the recycling of vitamin K, a vitamin critical to the physiology of blood clotting. Warfarin acts through a pathway that includes the Vitamin K Epoxide Reductase Complex (VKORC). The ability

Scientific Approach Panel 6.1
Personalized therapy for cystic fibrosis patients: the ivacaftor story

In 2015, when Barack Obama was the president of the United States, he highlighted the development of personalized medicine in his annual state-of-the-union speech; citing the success of a drug, called ivacaftor, used to treat some cystic fibrosis (CF) patients.

CF is a life-limiting autosomal recessive multi-system genetic disease. It is particularly characterized by thick mucus secretions in the airways and progressive lung damage, which is associated with respiratory tract infections that become increasingly difficult to treat.

The effectiveness and clinical utility of the new therapy, ivacaftor, was demonstrated in small, double blind, randomized controlled trials (RCTs) carried out between 2011 and 2015, in subgroups of CF patients, selected for particular mutant genotypes.

CF is caused by mutations to the CF transmembrane conductance regulator (**CFTR**) gene; patients are either homozygous or compound heterozygous for mutations with varying pathogenic effects. The wild type protein is located at the surface of epithelial cells that produce mucus, sweat, and digestive enzymes. The CFTR protein is an ion channel that regulates the transport of chloride ions and the movement of water into and out of the cell. An impaired ion channel causes mucus and other secretions to be too thick for normal physiology.

Nearly 2,000 different *CFTR* alleles have been identified in CF patients, some of which are common founder mutations and some of which are private mutations. The disease is subclassified according to the functional impact of the underlying genetic variants. Some deleterious mutations affect the expression level or stability of the CFTR protein; other mutations have an impact on its transport to the surface of the epithelial cell, or its function once it reaches the cell membrane. Approximately 4 per cent of CF patients worldwide have a missense mutation referred to as p.G551D, and the functional impact of the amino acid substitution of aspartic acid for glycine, is a conformational change in the CFTR protein and 'gating' defects in the opening of the ion channel. The small molecule, ivacaftor, supports the opening of the channel and enhances chloride ion secretion in patients with at least one of these mutations, and in some other patients who carry similar gating mutations.

The outcomes monitored in the ivacaftor RCTs included a lung function measurement, called the forced expiratory volume in one second (FEV_1). After just two weeks of treatment, there was improvement in the FEV_1 measurements for the participants who had been randomized to the experimental/test arms of the trial. In some of the RCTs, ivacaftor treatment was also associated with a reduction in the signs of progressive lung damage over a longer period of time. In these trials and in subsequent observational studies, ivacaftor was a supplementary therapy, used in combination with standard CF therapies such as antibiotic administration and pancreatic enzyme support.

In 2015, President Obama said 'I want the country that eliminated polio and mapped the human genome to lead a new era of medicine: one that delivers the right treatment at the right time. In some patients with cystic fibrosis, this approach has reversed a disease once thought unstoppable.'

Ivacaftor is licensed in the United States by the Food and Drug Administration (FDA) and in Europe by the European Medicines Agency (EMA). It was the first licensed therapy to target one of the underlying molecular defects that causes CF.

of VKORC to bind warfarin is modified by polymorphisms in the *VKORC1* gene. Some variants result in a quantitative reduction of mRNA and protein levels; other variants affect the catalytic domains of the protein. Identification of these genetic variants, and understanding their influence on protein expression and structure, allows us to make predictions about the oral anticoagulant effect of warfarin in individuals and to guide individual dosing decisions.

Many biomarkers are in clinical use for particular gene-drug combinations, and some important examples are listed in Table 6.1. In each case, an associated biomarker can provide useful information to improve patient outcomes.

Table 6.1 Examples of pharmacogenetic biomarkers.

Gene	Drug	Biomarker	Phenotype
BCHE	Choline esters, e.g. suxamethonium chloride	Sequence analysis of the coding region	ADR
BCR-ABL	Imatinib, dasatanib	t(9;22)(q34.1;q11.21) translocation can be detected in tumour cells by cytogenetic and molecular genetic techniques	Efficacy of treatment for chronic myeloid leukaemia
CFTR	Ivacaftor	Targeted genotype testing for missense SNPs including CFTR p.G551D	Treatment stratification and improved lung function
DPYD	Fluorouracil, capecitabine, tegafur	Targeted genotype testing for SNPs	ADR with treatment of solid tumours
ERBB2	Trastuzumab, lapatinib	Over-expression of protein on tumour cells detected by immunocytochemistry	Efficacy for HER2 positive breast cancer
CYP2D6	Codeine, tramadol, tricyclic antidepressants	Targeted genotype testing for SNPs	Efficacy & ADR
CYP2C9	Clopidogrel, warfarin, phenytoin	Targeted genotype testing for SNPs	Efficacy & ADR
G6PD	Rasburicase, sulphonamides	Targeted genotype testing for SNPs or sequence analysis of the coding region	ADR
HLA-B	Carbamazepine, allopurinol, abacavir	Targeted genotype testing for SNPs	ADR hypersensitivity
VKORC1	Warfarin	Targeted genotype testing for SNPs	Efficacy & ADR

The phenotypes monitored are efficacy (measured by improved survival or symptom relief) or adverse drug reactions (ADRs), and the biomarkers are drug-specific rather than disease-specific. SNP = single nucleotide polymorphism.

Case Study 6.1
Genetic testing to guide dose modification for warfarin

Isaac, a sixty-year-old man, was diagnosed with atrial fibrillation and treated with warfarin to reduce the risk of a blood clot and serious clinical complications such as a stroke or a heart attack. Before he started treatment six months ago, Isaac's doctor confirmed his age, height, weight, African-American ancestry, and medication history.

A blood sample was also taken for a genetic trial that Isaac had signed up for; laboratory biomarker tests for two genes, *VKORC1* and *CYP2C9* were completed. Isaac's starting dose was calculated to be lower than average; it was determined using a clinical algorithm that combined information from his demographic data and the results of genetic tests.

Notes and Discussion Points

- Warfarin is the most commonly prescribed anti-coagulant worldwide and used to treat millions of people every year. For example, warfarin is prescribed for individuals who have heart arrhythmias, or who have suffered a heart attack or stroke, to prevent clotting (thromboembolic) events.
- Warfarin is very effective for preventing thromboembolic events, but side-effects, including haemorrhage, are common and can be life-threatening; accounting for a significant proportion of hospital admissions for ADRs.
- Establishing an optimal warfarin dose can be a challenge because many clinical and dietary factors contribute to variance in drug response, as well as genetic factors. Calibration of a personalized treatment plan sometimes requires monitoring and modification over many months.

- A clinical algorithm is used to calculate a personalized starting dose; this includes data on age, height, weight, ethnicity, and other medications. The use of biomarkers for SNP variants in the genes *VKORC1* and *CYP2C9* can provide additional data to refine the warfarin dose calculations.
- Variants in the *VKORC1* protein product affect warfarin pharmacodynamics.
- The liver enzyme encoded by *CYP2C9* metabolizes warfarin and other commonly prescribed medicines. Some *CYP2C9* SNPs result in low or absent enzyme expression thus affecting warfarin pharmacokinetics.

List the pros and cons of using these genetic biomarkers to contribute to prescribing decisions about warfarin.

6.3   Cancer and Companion Diagnostic Tests

Pharmacogenetic tests have been applied within the oncology clinic for many years. The pathogenesis of cancer is a multistep process associated with the accumulation of mutations. There are some known inherited germline mutations, but the most common changes are somatic mutations that may alter critical components of protein-signalling pathways within cells. The accumulation of mutations is largely random, and so individuals exhibit great variability in their cancer biology: tumours of apparently similar classifications can differ markedly in their genetics.

Our understanding of tumour biology has developed over several decades; the first causative genetic change in a particular cancer was identified as a biomarker in 1973. That cancer was chronic myeloid leukaemia (CML), and Janet Rowley noted a chromosomal biomarker for a translocation event that results in the fusion of two oncogenes, *BCR* on chromosome 22 and *ABL1* on chromosome 9. The biomarker is a shortened chromosome 22 and is known as the Philadelphia chromosome. The products of both genes have kinase enzyme activities, which means they can change the activity of other proteins through the addition of a phosphate group. The kinase activity of the *BCR/ABL* fusion gene product is constitutively active. This is in contrast to the normal ABL protein, which, because of its role in intracellular signalling and protein networks that affect cell proliferation, adhesion and migration, has highly regulated kinase activity. The mutation therefore results in altered intracellular signalling which leads to a number of phenotypes that are hallmarks of cancer cells. The notable phenotypes include enhanced cell proliferation, blocks in programmed cell death (apoptosis), and impaired adhesion of the mutated cells to the bone marrow stroma.

Cytogenetic or molecular genetic detection of the *BCR/ABL* mutation is always used to confirm a diagnosis of CML. An understanding of the disease

> CYP gene variants are introduced in Chapter 2 and discussed in 6.4 later in this chapter.

> Cancer genetics was introduced in Chapters 2 and 5

Figure 6.2 An illustration of the pharmacodynamic targets and pharmacokinetics of imatinib.

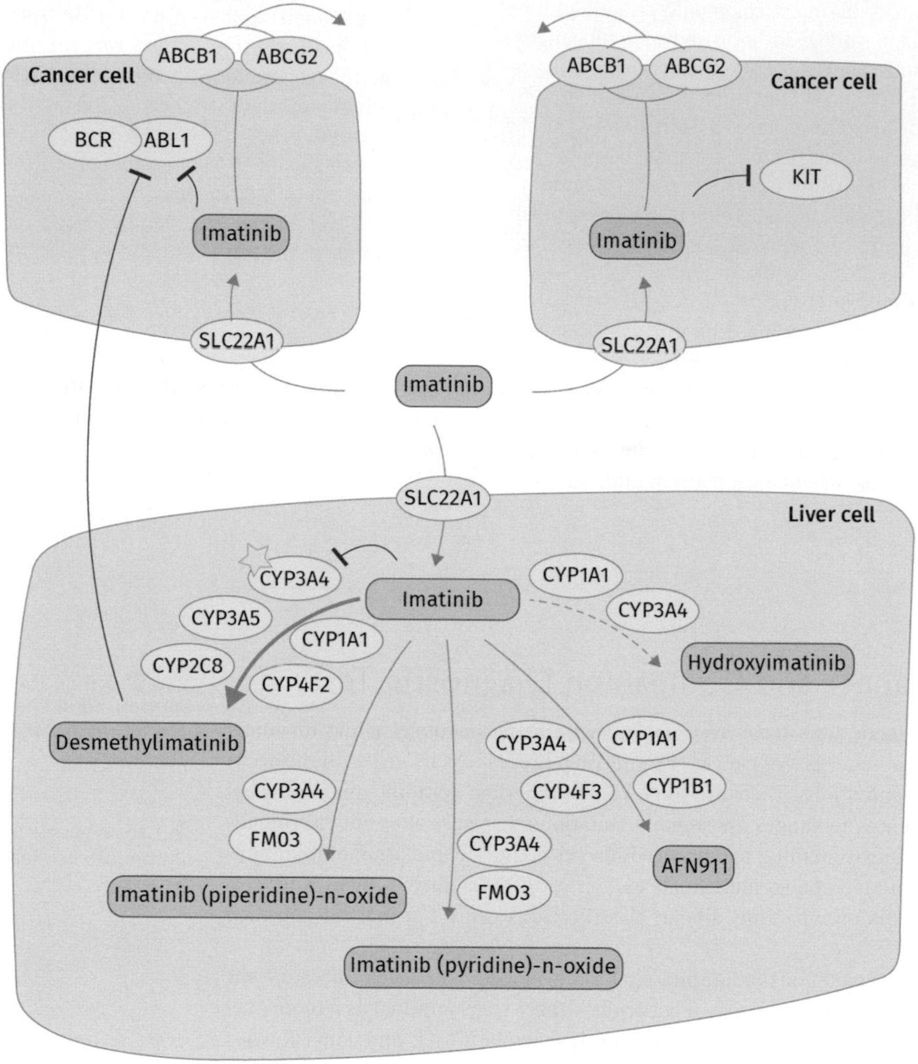

Image courtesy of PharmGKB / CC BY-SA 4.0.

biology led to the development of a rationally designed and highly effective new therapy in the late 1990s, known as the tyrosine kinase inhibitor, imatinib.

Several analytical methods are used to detect the *BCR/ABL* mutation; these include fluorescence *in situ* hybridization to detect the chromosome translocation or reverse transcriptase PCR to detect the fusion transcript. The biomarkers used to diagnose CML are known as companion diagnostic tests because a positive result is linked to a specific treatment protocol.

The scenario in Case Study 6.2 illustrates another classic example of a companion diagnostic test. Amplification of the *ERBB2* oncogene results in over-expression of one of the epidermal growth factor family of cell surface receptors called HER2. This mutation is associated with a poor prognosis in breast cancer; the protein activates intracellular signalling that increases the metastatic potential of tumour cells and inhibits apoptosis. The monoclonal antibody therapy, trastuzumab,

Case Study 6.2
The use of companion diagnostic tests to personalize treatment protocol

Maria is a seventy-four-year-old retired teacher. She was diagnosed with a breast carcinoma after noticing a small tethered lump in her left breast. She was treated surgically with a mastectomy, and is about to start chemotherapy and other medical management.

A biopsy of the tumour was analysed using immunohistochemistry for a number of tumour markers including **HER2 over-expression** (caused by amplification of the *ERBB2* oncogene). The histology report showed a moderate amount of expression of the protein in about 40 per cent of the tumour cells (and refers to score 3+ for an invasive ductal carcinoma).

The positive result from this companion diagnostic test means that Maria will receive the monoclonal antibody trastuzumab (Herceptin) as well as chemotherapeutic agents in her treatment regime.

Notes and Discussion Points

- Immunohistochemistry is an important diagnostic laboratory technique that is particularly useful for subclassifying diseases such as breast cancer.
- Sections of stained tissue are analysed using microscopy. Antibodies are used to localize specific protein epitopes or antigens, and the position of binding, within the tissue section and individual cells, is visualized using a variety of staining protocols. See Figure 6.3, taking note of the brown staining of the cell membranes where the HER2 protein is over-expressed in the tumour cells.

Figure 6.3 Immunohistochemistry analysis using formalin-fixed, paraffin-embedded breast tissue biopsy. The HER2 score is 3+. The magnification is x200.

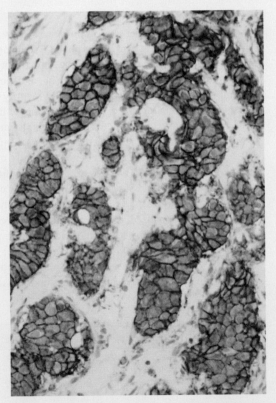

Image courtesy of Dr Joseph Murphy, Consultant Histopathologist at the Norfolk and Norwich University Hospital.

- The microscopic observations of HER2 anti- body staining are scored in a systematic way to aid treatment stratification; see Table 6.2 for a typical protocol for systematic interpretation

of the data. Clinical trials have shown that pa- tients with positive results will benefit most from treatment with the monoclonal antibody trastuzumab.

Table 6.2 An example of the protocol used to score the HER2 immunohistochemistry results.

Antibody Staining Observed	Biomarker Scoring	Overall Result (interpretation of HER-2 over-expression)
None or faint staining in < 10% tumour cells.	0	Negative
Faint staining in > 10% tumour cells but the cell membranes are not completely stained.	1+	Negative
Moderate & complete membrane staining in > 10% tumour cells.	2+	Equivocal or weakly positive
Strong & complete membrane staining in > 30% tumour cells.	3+	Strongly positive

is prescribed if protein over-expression is detected by immunocytochemistry in the routine histology testing of tumour samples. Trastuzumab binds to the extracellular domain of the HER2 protein with a very high affinity and this leads to cytostatic and cytotoxic events; that is, less cell division and more cell death occurs.

Companion diagnostic tests are used to identify particular *actionable muta- tions*, which means there is a treatment available linked to the mutation or al- tered biochemical pathway detected. Actionable mutations are often the driver mutations that directly or indirectly confer a selective growth advantage to the cells, driving carcinogenesis. Cancers are usually categorized according to the organ and tissue affected but it is now proposed that signatures of somatic on- cogene mutations could serve as biomarkers that cut across traditional tissue- specific classifications; the identification of actionable mutations in this way can result in personalized, and therefore more effective, treatment regimes. For example, Figure 6.2 shows the pharmacodynamic pathways for imatinib. This drug is one example of a tyrosine kinase inhibitor; it was specifically designed to treat CML but it is also used to treat other tumour types (e.g. gastrointestinal tumours) with actionable variants of the same signalling pathway.

 Key Points

- Rational drug design has resulted from a detailed understanding of the genetic cause and pathophysiology of many types of cancer.
- The clinical use of these drugs is informed by companion diagnostic labora- tory tests.

6.4   Pharmacokinetics and Adverse Drug Reactions (ADRs)

The term pharmacokinetics describes how the systems of the body handle a drug once it has been administered to an individual. It considers the **absorption** and **distribution** of the drug; the process of **metabolism** to produce both active metabolites and less-toxic, **excretable** metabolites; and ultimately the excretion of the drug or its products. The physiological processes highlighted above have led to a set of genes being defined by the acronym *ADME genes.*

The effort to define the key variants of the *ADME* genes that encode proteins for the *absorption, distribution, metabolism and excretion* of medicines is demonstrated by the vast body of curated information presented in the Pharmacogenomics Knowledgebase. This publicly accessible resource is managed by Stanford University and it appraises published research about pharmacogenetics and stratified medicine. Its curators annotate important genetic variants and pharmacogenetic pathways. Its clinical information includes drug-dosing guidelines and it identifies a group of genes as *Very Important Pharmacogenes (VIPs)* because there are clinically actionable biomarkers associated with them. Some of the *VIP* genes listed are members of the cytochrome P450 (CYP) liver enzyme superfamily.

> ### 💡 Key Points
>
> - The term pharmacokinetics describes a drug's metabolism, including uptake; conversion to active metabolites; breakdown; and excretion. It can also be described as *what the body does to the drug.*

Figure 6.4 An illustration of the curated data on a VIP gene (CYP2D6) webpage from the Pharmacogenomics Knowledgebase.

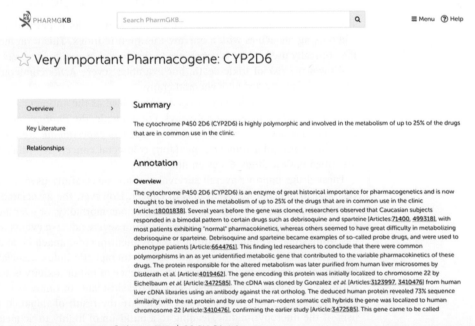

Particular CYP enzymes are highly polymorphic within populations. The enzymes encoded by the genes *CYP2D6* and *CYP2D9* metabolize many of our commonly prescribed medicines including warfarin, antidepressants, and analgesics. The plasma concentration of a drug (or its metabolites) can vary significantly between patients because of heterogeneity in enzyme activity, which in turn can be predicted by genetic tests for underlying polymorphisms, from missense SNVs to truncating null mutations.

In some situations, patients can be classified as ultra-metabolizers, and will gain little efficacy from their medicine because plasma concentrations of the drug remain low if the active drug is rapidly metabolized and excreted. Conversely, in situations where toxic drug metabolites can build up, the risk of adverse effects is actually greater in the ultra-metabolizers who carry genetic variants that result in higher enzyme activities. This is demonstrated in some children receiving the pro-drug codeine, which becomes quickly metabolized to morphine, causing opioid-induced respiratory depression.

> which are discussed in Chapter 2.

A crude form of pharmacogenetics has been applied in clinical practice for some time because we know that certain genetic variants involved in drug metabolism are more prevalent in populations from some parts of the world than others. We see ethnic variation in the frequency of particular alleles, such as SNPs of the *CYP2D6* gene. These ancestral differences mean that the usefulness of a particular biomarker may be population-specific. For example, more than a quarter of Ethiopians are *CYP2D6* ultra-metabolizers. Knowledge about the high frequency of particular alleles in this ancestral group already influences cautious prescribing decisions for drugs metabolized via this pathway. However, precise biomarkers for the functional variants would be particularly useful in this context. There is a danger that certain drug options are abandoned because of common side effects for some populations. Instead of applying this blunt epidemiological instrument for individual prescribing decisions, a specific genetic test would be more useful to guide treatment within a healthcare system.

6.5   Considering the Narrow Therapeutic Index

The case for using genetic tests to prevent severe ADRs is particularly strong when using medicines with a narrow therapeutic index. This term means that the clinically useful dose is very close to the dose that results in severe toxicity, and even the risk of toxic death. For example, severe ADRs commonly affect cancer patients treated with chemotherapy.

One class of chemotherapy drugs is categorized as the antimetabolites; these disrupt fundamental cellular pathways. For example, the *fluoropyrimidines* target folate metabolism. *Fluoropyrimidines* such as *capecitabine* are used worldwide for many solid tumours, including colorectal cancer. See Mikkel's story, described in Case Study 6.3 as an illustration.

These drugs improve overall survival and are successfully used to cure cancers and to manage the symptoms of cancer. However, the associated adverse effects of this chemotherapy can result in serious morbidity, or even mortality: approximately one fifth of patients suffer from severe adverse events including gastrointestinal symptoms, cardiac toxicity, neutropenia, anaemia, and abnormal liver function tests. In fact, the narrow therapeutic index associated with the use of *fluoropyrimidines* means that evidence of minor toxicity is associated with favourable clinical responses such as the shrinkage of tumours.

A significant proportion of severe ADRs are the result of impaired metabolism of the fluoropyrimidine, leading to a build-up of highly toxic metabolites.

Case Study 6.3
An adverse drug reaction (ADR) with chemotherapy

Mikkel is a fifty-seven-year-old man undergoing treatment for a stage 3 colorectal carcinoma at a cancer centre in England. His primary tumour and a blood sample were analysed using whole genome sequencing as part of a national genomics research project, but data about the somatic genetic profile of his tumour, and his drug metabolizing genetic profile, were not ready when he started an adjuvant chemotherapy protocol. He took capecitabine twice daily for twelve days of his first twenty-one-day treatment cycle. However, he was told to delay his next dose because he reported diarrhoea and an oral infection to the specialist nurse who regularly rang him at home. Mikkel's symptoms got progressively worse and he was admitted to hospital on day fourteen of the cycle, with very severe diarrhoea, fever, and life-threatening failure of his bone marrow, which meant that he had a very low number of leukocytes in his blood.

Mikkel was admitted to the intensive care unit because he developed signs of sepsis. He made a gradual recovery after optimal treatment and supportive care, and returned home 18 days after his hospital admission. Mikkel had suffered a life-threatening ADR and genetic tests show he carries a variant that causes DPD deficiency. For cases like Mikkel's, the dose of capecitabine and some other similar drugs used should be significantly reduced because of slow drug metabolism and clearance.

Notes and Discussion Points

1. Early in the twentieth century, the scientist and clinician Lucy Wills identified folate as an essential micronutrient. Folate-dependent metabolism was subsequently found to be critical for cell division because it is essential for DNA biosynthesis, DNA repair, and DNA methylation. Therefore, rapidly dividing cells are particularly sensitive to deficiencies in folate and/or its metabolism. This makes folate metabolism an effective target for drugs used in the treatment of cancer and chronic inflammatory disease, which are characterized by rapid cell turnover. Fluoropyrimidines such as capecitabine interfere with folate metabolism and are very effective cancer therapies. However, they have a toxic impact on rapidly dividing normal tissues as well as the targeted cancer cells.

2. Toxicity from capecitabine can be particularly significant for epithelial cells in the skin and gastrointestinal system, and the bone marrow. Approximately 20 per cent of patients suffer from severe ADRs including diarrhoea and vomiting: leading to dehydration, low numbers of blood cells (neutropenia, anaemia, and thrombocytopenia) and abnormal liver function tests. Starting doses are usually based on the age, sex, and body mass index of the patient; and patients are closely monitored for evidence of toxicity once treatment starts. If severe ADRs occur the chemotherapy is suspended (either temporarily or permanently) which can affect clinical outcomes and even survival.

3. Some of the heritability of these ADRs is explained by genetic variants (including exon-skipping and missense SNVs) in the *DPYD* gene that encodes the key pharmacokinetic catabolic enzyme for fluoropyrimidines, DPD. The variants can serve as biomarkers for a risk of ADRs and doses can be modified accordingly (see Figure 6.5).

How could pharmacogenetic tests have improved Mikkel's experience?

Dihydropyrimidine dehydrogenase (DPD) is the key liver enzyme that usually catabolizes most of the drug into non-cytotoxic metabolites. However, the activity of DPD varies widely between patients and some people have complete enzyme deficiency. *DPYD* is the gene that encodes DPD and it is highly polymorphic between individuals, and some people are homozygous for rare, 'catalytically inactive' *DPYD* alleles. The association between these variants and toxicity is very well-established and the use of genetic biomarkers to guide the dosing of *fluoropyrimidines* has been recommended but is not always used in clinical practice.

Figure 6.5 An illustration of how the starting dose of capecitabine can be modified to reduce ADRs.

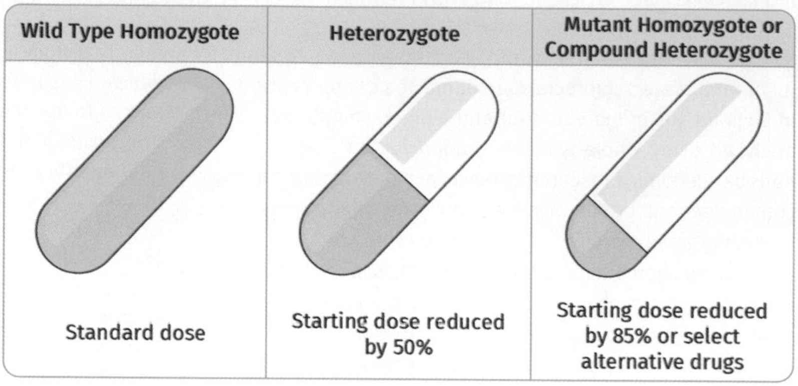

Wild Type Homozygote	Heterozygote	Mutant Homozygote or Compound Heterozygote
Standard dose	Starting dose reduced by 50%	Starting dose reduced by 85% or select alternative drugs

6.6   Rare Hypersensitivity Reactions

Severe idiosyncratic hypersensitivity reactions are particularly dangerous ADRs that have been associated with specific genetic variants in susceptible individuals. These very rare events are mediated by the immune system, and not linked to the measurable pharmacokinetic or pharmacodynamic parameters described. Severe skin reactions and liver damage are the usual manifestations and they can result in life-threatening conditions—for example, drug-induced liver injury and toxic epidermal necrolysis.

 in 6.2 and 6.4

 with discussions of biomarkers in Chapters 2 and 3

Predictive **biomarkers** are available for particular genetic variants of the human leukocyte antigen (HLA) system that are risk factors for these hypersensitivity reactions. Genetic testing can be used before starting therapy, to screen out susceptible individuals who carry the associated rare variants; so that they are not exposed to the risk of a particular drug. This approach is used clinically when prescribing antiretroviral drugs such as abacavir, or when prescribing carbamazepine for the treatment of seizures.

It is worth noting though that the frequency of the *HLA* B*1502 allele, which is implicated in carbamazepine hypersensitivity, ranges from about 8 per cent in Thailand to 0.1 per cent in populations of other ancestries, including European populations. Therefore, this is likely to be a valuable predictive biomarker in Thailand, but will be much less useful in European populations.

Key Points

• Severe hypersensitivity disorders can be fatal. Rare *HLA* alleles associated with abacavir ADRs are tested for routinely.

6.7   Clinical Validity, Clinical Utility, and Ethical Considerations

It is worth considering why pharmacogenetic testing is still rarely used in the clinic despite the association of so many well-characterized predictive biomarkers with drug response phenotypes.

In their favour, nearly all pharmacogenetic tests for particular mutations are very reliable in the laboratory. In other words, their **analytic validity** is very high because the DNA tests accurately predict the presence or absence of a given marker.

However, different factors affect how reliably a given biomarker can predict the presence or absence of a drug response; that is, their **clinical validity** is variable.

First, the predictive value of a biomarker will depend on both the frequency of the event of interest (how common is the ADR or what proportion of patients have a beneficial response), and the prevalence of the associated genetic marker. As we saw in 6.4, 'Pharmacokinetics and Adverse Drug Reactions (ADRs)', ethnicity will affect allele frequencies within a given population; therefore, the detection of particular *CYP2D6* alleles is useful in Ethiopian populations to detect ultra-metabolizers because the associated allele frequency is high in this ancestral group.

Second, to use biomarkers to stratify treatment decisions, we need to consider the discrimination profile for the biomarker, and the concepts of test sensitivity and specificity. The sensitivity of any test refers to its ability to correctly identify those individuals *with* the phenotype of interest; the specificity of the test is its ability to correctly identify those *without* the phenotype.

An illustration of an optimal, and also a typical, discrimination profile of a pharmacogenetic biomarker test is shown in Figure 6.6.

Perfect diagnostic tests would have no overlap in the spectrum of positive and negative tests; in reality the sensitivity of a test is improved at the cost of specificity and vice versa.

In ideal circumstances, any pharmacogenetic biomarker would reliably separate out two contrasting groups of patients: (1) those likely to derive considerable benefit from their treatment and few ADRs; and (2) those with poor benefit: harm ratio (limited response with high likelihood of ADRs; see Figure 6.7). In practice, many drugs have a narrow therapeutic index (for example, warfarin and cancer chemotherapy), so most individuals who gain benefit from their treatment also encounter ADRs.

Pharmacogenetic tests have been assumed to carry fewer ethical concerns than other predictive clinical genetic tests. This is because the tests are specific

Figure 6.6 Discrimination profiles for a biomarker for a continuous trait. This biomarker is to detect ADR risk, which is associated with a low metabolic enzyme activity. (a) Profile for an optimal biomarker. In this profile, there is a clear separation of true positive (TP) and true negative (TN) test results. (b) Profile for a typical, real-world example. There is considerable overlap in the test spectrum, resulting in high rates of false negative and false positive results for the biomarker.

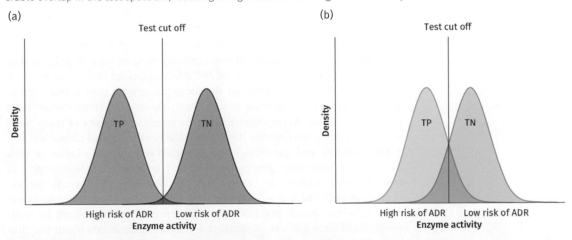

This illustration is based on ideas described by Soreide, Kjetil (2009). *Journal of Clinical Pathology*, 62(1), 1–5.

Figure 6.7 Treatment stratification and pharmacogenetic testing. An illustration of four theoretical phenotype groups that biomarker panels might identify.

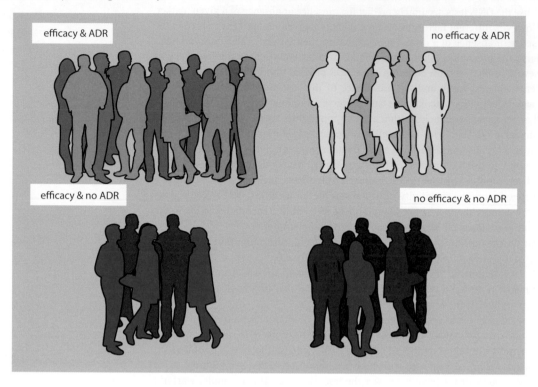

for a particular medication only, and there are rarely implications, from test results, for other family members or indeed any social consequences for the treated individual. However, some biomarkers carry a risk that stratifying the patient group could result in a form of genetic discrimination. Some patients will be refused access to an expensive new drug because they are not predicted to gain as much benefit as another group of patients—even though they would perhaps gain some benefit. A patient finding themselves in the 'molecularly un-stratified' group for a new precision therapy can mean that a therapeutic route associated with hope is shut down for the patient; which is a particularly potent concern for the oncology clinic where there may be few curative options.

Finally, the genetic variation identified by the biomarker may be one of several contributory factors for a given outcome; reducing the sensitivity of the biomarker. For example, if we consider the use of *DPYD* biomarkers for patients treated with fluoropyrimidines the sensitivity of the individual genetic tests is low because many genetic variants contribute to both pharmacokinetic and pharmacodynamic pathways (for example, see Figure 6.8); so the genetic complexity of many pharmacogenetic traits compromises the clinical validity of individual biomarkers.

❯ see 6.5 'Considering the Narrow Therapeutic Index'

The sensitivity and specificity of an individual test, a panel of tests, or even data derived from whole genome analysis may be impressive, but the goal in medicine is to improve the clinical outcomes that are important to the patient. Ultimately, the real-world value of genetic tests for both individuals and for populations within healthcare systems can only be determined by well-controlled clinical trials. In 2019, there is still insufficient data about the clinical utility of many of these promising pharmacogenetics tests; which means

Figure 6.8 An illustration of the pharmacodynamic and pharmacokinetic pathways for the fluoropyrimidines including capecitabine. (a) The cellular targets are shown for the metabolites of three commonly prescribed fluoropyrimidines, tegafur, fluorouracil, and capecitabine. These chemotherapy drugs interfere with the essential metabolic processes illustrated; folate metabolism, nucleic acid synthesis, DNA repair, and apoptosis. PK: pharmacokinetic. (b) The metabolism of tegafur, fluorouracil, and capecitabine in a liver cell is illustrated. The drugs and their metabolites are illustrated by the purple boxes PD: pharmacodynamic.

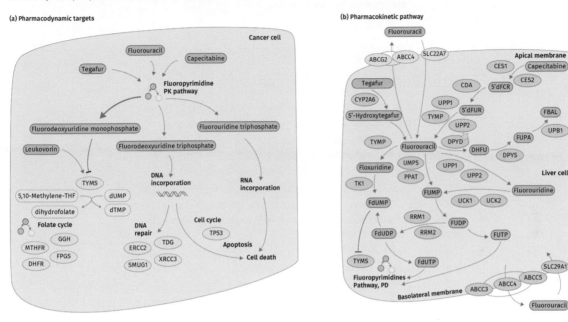

Image courtesy of PharmGKB/CC BY-SA 4.0.

we don't actually know that the tests will provide useful information that can improve patient outcomes and not cause unintended harm.

6.8   From Pharmacogenetics to Pharmacogenomics

The individual pharmacogenetic biomarkers described in this chapter have been integrated into routine clinical practice, or have the potential to be actionable biomarkers.

However, most of these pharmacogenetic traits are polygenic (or multifactorial) and there is an expectation that a wider pharmaco*genomic* approach to testing will improve the predictive value of the tests. Increasingly, panels of ADME gene variants are tested in parallel to improve the test sensitivity and, as whole genome sequencing becomes more widespread, additional variants of interest will be identified.

In the United States and in Europe, research centres have been established to facilitate the routine clinical implementation of pharmacogenomics. They have identified the central importance of integrated electronic medical records to:

1. embed actionable pharmacogenetic data such as particular CYP variants into an individual's medical records; and to use laboratory reports that are clear: avoiding complex genetic or pharmacological terminology;

2. support the use of genomic prescribing systems that generate electronic prescriptions tailored to an individual's genotype.

Having access to genetic data within medical records is proposed, because clinicians can't always delay prescribing decisions to wait for genetic testing to be completed. Digital infrastructure, such as the use of electronic prescribing systems that use algorithms informed by genetic data, will also combat some of the current barriers to the implementation of pharmacogenetic tests within mainstream health services.

Chapter Summary

- Pharmacogenetics and pharmacogenomics is the analysis of the interaction between an individual's genes or genome and drug responses.

- Pharmacodynamics describes the interaction between a drug and its molecular target or *what the drug does to the body*. Pharmacokinetics describes a drug's metabolism or *what the body does to the drug*.

- The use of individualized treatment protocols that depend on this genetic data is often described as *personalized medicine* or and even as *precision medicine*, but the differences observed in response to most medicines are complex and not fully defined.

- The biomarkers described in this chapter can provide some probabilistic information about the efficacy, dosage requirements, or ADRs that an individual patient might have with a given drug.

- The use of personalized medicine is already well-established in the oncology clinic. The design of new and effective biological therapies has resulted from a detailed understanding of the genetic cause and pathophysiology of many types of cancer. The clinical use of these drugs is often informed by companion diagnostic genetic tests.

- Data about the biomarkers can be collected from tests of individual loci and gene panels, or from whole genome analysis.

Further Reading

Review:

Pharmacogenomics (2019) Dan Roden, *et al.* Lancet; 394: 521-532 doi: 10.1016/S0140-6736(19)31276-0 A review that underlines and elaborates on the themes from this chapter and book.

Book:

Dudley, J. T. and Karczewski, K. J. (2013). *Exploring personal genomics*. Oxford: Oxford University Press.

Discussion Questions

6.1 See Case Study 6.1, and list the pros and cons of using these genetic biomarkers to contribute to prescribing decisions about warfarin.

6.2 See Case Study 6.3, and consider how pharmacogenetic tests could have improved the patient's experience.

GLOSSARY

1000 Genomes Project An international research project that began in 2008 to establish a detailed catalogue of human genetic variation. See www.internationalgenome.org/1000-genomes-project-publications

Adenine A nitrogen-containing purine base found in DNA and RNA.

Allele A variant form of a particular gene.

Alternative splicing A regulatory mechanism in gene expression. Different forms of messenger RNAs and protein isoforms can be generated from the same gene.

Amniocentesis A sampling procedure to aspirate amniotic fluid and cells (amniocytes) that are used for prenatal diagnosis.

Amplification A type of mutation and a cancer genetic term. A genetic alteration/mutation that results in many copies of a small (< a few megabases) DNA segment of the genome.

Analytic validity The analytic validity of a genetic test is its ability to measure accurately and reliably the variant/s of interest.

Anaphase lag Delayed movement of a chromosome or chromatid to the poles of a cell during the anaphase stage of cell division. It can lead to chromosome loss and monosomy.

Aneuploidy An abnormal number of chromosomes in a cell.

Antagonist A molecule, e.g. a drug, that stops the action or effect of another molecule.

Anticipation For some genetic conditions, the signs and symptoms tend to become more severe and appear at an earlier age as the condition is passed from one generation to the next.

Apoptosis Programmed cell death; in response to a stimulus, a pathway is triggered that leads to the destruction of the cell by a characteristic set of reactions.

Autosomal dominant Autosomal dominance is a pattern of inheritance characteristic of some genetic diseases. 'Autosomal' means that the gene in question is located on one of the numbered, or non-sex, chromosomes. 'Dominant' means that a single copy of the disease-associated mutation is enough to cause the disease.

Autosomal recessive Autosomal recessive is a pattern of inheritance characteristic of some genetic diseases. 'Autosomal' means that the gene in question is located on one of the numbered, or non-sex, chromosomes. 'Recessive' means two copies of the mutation are needed to cause the disease.

Autosome One of the chromosomes that are not the sex chromosomes X or Y. Humans have twenty-two pairs of autosomes and one pair of sex chromosomes (the X and Y). Autosomes are numbered roughly in relation to their sizes. That is, chromosome 1 has approximately 2,800 gene loci, while chromosome 22 has approximately 750 genes.

B-form of DNA The DNA double helix can have different conformations called A-, B-, or Z-forms. The double helix of the B-form (which is the most prevalent form in nature) was revealed by Rosalind Franklin and Raymond Gosling using X-ray crystallography. A famous image was produced for the diffraction pattern generated. This image is often referred to as Photograph 51 in the research literature.

Bioinformatic pipeline A series of computational steps to translate the nucleotide sequence of the DNA sample into a clinically actionable result. Software is used to organize, analyse, and interpret data.

Bioinformatics The computerized integration of mathematical and statistical methods to analyse molecular data that is produced from genome, transcriptome, and proteome analysis.

Biomarker A factor that can be objectively measured and evaluated as an indicator of normal biological processes, pathogenic processes, or pharmacological response.

Codon A codon is a trinucleotide sequence of DNA or RNA that corresponds to a specific amino acid. The genetic code describes the relationship between the sequence of DNA bases (A, C, G, and T) in a gene and the corresponding protein sequence that it encodes. The cell reads the sequence of the gene in groups of three bases. There are sixty-four different codons: sixty-one specify amino acids while the remaining three are used as stop signals.

Clinical validity The accuracy with which a test identifies a particular phenotype such as disease status.

Companion diagnostic test A specific diagnostic test that is used to guide the selection of a particular treatment.

Compound heterozygote Carrying two different mutations in homologous copies of a gene.

Congenital abnormalities Any abnormality that is present at birth. The cause may or may not be genetic.

Congenital Adrenal Hyperplasia (CAH) Congenital adrenal hyperplasia is an inherited condition present from birth (congenital).

The adrenal gland is larger than usual (hyperplasia). It is described as an inborn error of metabolism because the body is missing a normal copy of an enzyme that stimulates the adrenal glands to release the cortisol hormone.

Consanguinity Genetic relatedness between individuals who are descendants of at least one recent common ancestor.

Copy number variant (CNV) A genetic variant that arises from the gain or loss of very large segments of DNA to and from the genome.

CRISPR CRISPR is an abbreviation of Clustered Regularly Interspaced Short Palindromic Repeats, which are part of a bacterial defence system. The term is also used for describing CRISPR-Cas9 genome editing technology, which comprises a guide RNA sequence and a nuclease enzyme that can introduce double strand breaks into DNA which will be repaired; specific sequence modifications can be made in conjunction with this approach.

CYP (Cytochrome P450) family A highly polymorphic family of phase I enzymes (important for the liver metabolism of prescribed drugs and other compounds). One protein encoded by the gene *CYP2D6* metabolizes ~ 25 per cent of all prescribed drugs and about seventy different genetic variants (alleles) have been described. There is inter-ethnic variation in the allele frequencies and while some alleles are associated with poor or no enzyme activity, others result in very high rates of drug metabolism and so low plasma concentration of prescribed drugs.

Cystic fibrosis and *CFTR* Cystic fibrosis (CF) is an inherited disease which mainly affects the lungs and digestive system. These organs are impaired with thick, sticky mucus which can lead to symptoms like a cough, chest infections and difficulty absorbing and digesting fat in food; it is a multi-system disorder that results in a general failure to thrive. It is often described as an inborn error of metabolism because the body is missing a normal copy of a protein encoded by the *CFTR* gene which

lies on chromosome 7. The encoded protein, the cystic fibrosis transmembrane conductance regulator (CFTR) is responsible for regulation of sodium, chloride, and bicarbonate transport in many tissues of the body.

Cytosine A nitrogen-containing pyrimidine base found in DNA and RNA.

Deciphering Developmental Disorders (DDD) A UK study to advance clinical genetic practice for children with developmental disorders (www.ddduk.org).

***De novo* mutation** A new, rather than inherited, mutation.

Diploid genome Diploid is a cell or organism that has paired chromosomes, one from each parent. In humans, cells (other than human sex cells) are usually diploid and have twenty-three pairs of chromosomes. Human sex cells (egg and sperm cells) contain a single set of chromosomes and are known as haploid.

Direct-to-consumer genetic tests Some companies provide people with access to their genetic information without the intervention of a healthcare provider or health insurance company in the process. The tests provided commercially are often for markers related to increased disease risk and ancestry or genealogy testing. DNA is usually extracted from saliva or mouth swab samples for these tests.

DNA (Deoxyribose nucleic acid) The DNA molecule consists of two strands that wind around one another to form a double helix. Each strand has a backbone made of alternating sugar (deoxyribose) and phosphate groups. Attached to each sugar is one of four bases: adenine (A), cytosine (C), guanine (G), or thymine (T). The two strands are held together by bonds between the bases; adenine bonds with thymine, and cytosine bonds with guanine. The sequence of the bases along the backbones serves as instructions for assembling protein and RNA molecules.

DNA hybridization The annealing of a single stranded DNA molecule to a complementary DNA sequence.

DNA ligases Enzymes that join two DNA molecules together via phosphodiester bonds. The process is energy-dependent.

DNA polymerases Enzymes that synthesize DNA molecules from nucleotide building blocks. These enzymes are essential for DNA replication.

DNA sequencing DNA sequencing is a laboratory technique used to determine the exact sequence of bases (A, C, G, and T) in a DNA molecule. The DNA base sequence carries the information a cell needs to assemble protein and RNA molecules. DNA sequence information is important to scientists investigating the functions of genes. The technology of DNA sequencing was made faster and less expensive as a part of the Human Genome Project.

DNA synthesis DNA synthesis or replication is the process by which a molecule of DNA is duplicated. When a cell divides, it must first duplicate its genome so that each daughter cell has a complete set of chromosomes. The in vivo process is copied in the laboratory as part of many molecular genetic methods; e.g. in the polymerase chain reaction and DNA sequencing.

Driver mutation A cancer genetic term; a mutation that directly or indirectly confers a selective growth advantage to the cell in which it occurs.

Dysmorphism Abnormal physical appearance.

ENCODE An encyclopedia of DNA Elements (and a research programme). It was established to identify all functional elements in the human and mouse genomes: see www.encodeproject.org

Epigenetics and epigenetic changes Heritable changes caused by the activation and deactivation of genes without any change in the underlying DNA sequence of the organism. The word epigenetics is of Greek origin and literally means over and above (*epi*) the genome.

Variations in gene expression that are not caused by changes in the DNA sequence but do include chemical modifications to chromatin and DNA, such as methylation. DNA molecules are methylated by the addition of a methyl group to carbon position 5 on cytosine bases that are positioned adjacent to a guanine base (CpG sites). Transcription is usually repressed by DNA methylation and histone de-acetylation. Epigenetic modifications during tumorigenesis can lead to the wrong gene being switched on or off, for the given physiological circumstances, or for the given tissue type.

Epistasis Epistasis describes gene–gene interactions. The expression of one gene is affected by the expression of one or more independently inherited genes.

Euchromatin Extended and more transcriptionally active region of a chromosome.

Exon An exon is the portion of a gene that codes for amino acids. Most human gene sequences are broken up by one or more DNA sequences called introns. The parts of the gene sequence that are expressed in the protein are called exons, because they are expressed, while the parts of the gene sequence that are not expressed in the protein are called introns, because they come in between the exons.

Expressivity Variation in the type and severity of the phenotype associated with a particular genetic variant or genotype.

Flip-tip inversion A structural variant of the *F8* gene that causes severe cases of Haemophilia A.

Fluorescence *in situ* hybridization (FISH) Fluorescence *in situ* hybridization (FISH) is a laboratory technique for detecting and locating a specific DNA sequence on a chromosome. The technique relies on exposing chromosomes to a small DNA sequence called a probe that has a fluorescent molecule attached to it. The probe sequence binds to its corresponding sequence on the chromosome.

Founder effect The founder effect is the reduction in genetic variation that results when a small subset of a large population is used to establish a new colony. The new population may be very different from the original population, both in terms of its genotypes and phenotypes. Founder members of particular new populations may be carriers of mutant alleles for some traits (recessive or late-onset dominant) and so within that population these alleles are at a higher frequency than in the wider population.

Founder mutation A genetic variation observed at high frequency in a group that is or was geographically or culturally isolated, in which one or more of the ancestors was a carrier of the altered gene.

Frameshift mutation The addition or loss of DNA bases that changes the reading frame of a gene, caused by insertions, deletions, and duplications of bases.

Gene A linear DNA sequence that can produce a functional RNA molecule. Most genes encode a polypeptide sequence.

Gene panel Genetic tests that analyse multiple genes simultaneously for variants that may be associated with a disease phenotype. Also called multi-gene test and multiple-gene test.

Genetic architecture The underlying genetic basis of a phenotype or trait. Refers to the number and the effect sizes of the individual loci that contribute to the phenotype.

Genetic counselling The use of genetic counselling steps should be a non-directive and non-judgemental method to pass on appropriate factual information.

Genocopy The same phenotype or trait caused by a different genotype.

Genome The genome is the entire set of genetic instructions found in a cell. In humans, the genome consists of twenty-three pairs of chromosomes, found in the nucleus, as well as a small DNA complement found in the cells' mitochondria. Each set of twenty-three chromosomes contains approximately 3.1 billion base pairs of DNA sequence.

Genome-Wide Association Study (GWAS) A GWAS is a method or study design used in genetics research to associate specific genetic variations with particular diseases. It involves scanning the genomes from many different people and looking for genetic markers that can be used to predict the presence of a disease. Once such genetic markers are identified, they can be used to understand how genes contribute to the disease and develop better prevention and treatment strategies. The method involves the analysis of thousands or millions of polymorphic markers across the complete sets of DNA, or genomes, of many people to find genetic variations associated with a particular disease. Typically, the genetic results from research participants with a defined disease are compared with the genetic results from a matched control cohort.

Germline mutation A gene change in a reproductive cell (egg or sperm) that becomes incorporated into the DNA of every cell in the body of the offspring. A variant contained within the germline can be passed from parent to offspring, and is, therefore, hereditary.

Giemsa A laboratory staining chemical which can be used to define and differentiate cellular and chromosome structure (referred to as G-banding). It is used in cytogenetics, histopathology, and in laboratory haematology.

Guanine A nitrogen-containing purine base found in DNA and RNA.

Haploid A cell or organism having a single set of chromosomes. Sexually reproducing organisms are diploid (having two sets of chromosomes, one from each parent). In humans, there are twenty-three chromosomes in a diploid set, egg and sperm (germ) cells are haploid.

Haploinsufficiency Loss of one copy of a gene, e.g. because of a deletion or other loss-of-function mutation, leaves a single functional copy of a gene in a diploid cell or organism. Having only one copy of the wild-type allele may not be sufficient because the gene product will be approximately half of the normal level.

HapMap HapMap (short for 'haplotype map') is the name of the International HapMap Project, a project that relates variations in human DNA sequences with genes associated with health. A haplotype is a set of DNA variations, or polymorphisms, that tend to be inherited together. A haplotype can refer to a combination of alleles or to a set of single nucleotide polymorphisms (SNPs) found on the same chromosome. The HapMap describes common patterns of genetic variation among people.

Hardy–Weinberg equilibrium This is a term and a mathematical formula used in population genetics. Godfrey Hardy and Wilhelm Weinberg described a mathematical model for the distribution of genotypes in a stable population.

The binomial equation $(p^2 + 2pq + q^2 = 1)$ is often used to determine expected genotype frequencies. p and q represent the frequencies of two alternative alleles in a population, and their frequencies add up to 1.

Helicase An enzyme that unwinds two annealed DNA strands in a process requiring energy.

Hemizygous A cell or individual with a single copy of a gene instead of the usual two copies. The genes of the male X chromosome are hemizygous.

Hereditary information (in humans) This is the information contained in the genes/DNA found in the human chromosomes and mitochondria. This information is passed from one generation (of cells and individuals) to the next generation.

Heredity The passing of genetic information and characteristics from parents to offspring.

Heritability The proportion of the variance of a characteristic that is attributable to genetic factors.

Heterochromatin Unusually condensed and transcriptionally inactive region of a chromosome.

Heteroplasmy The presence of more than one type of mitochondrial genome within the cell or individual.

Heterozygote/ous Heterozygous refers to having inherited different forms of a particular gene from each parent. A heterozygous genotype stands in contrast to a homozygous genotype, where an individual inherits identical forms of a particular gene from each parent.

Heterozygote advantage For some conditions, having one mutated copy of a gene in each cell is advantageous and improves reproductive fitness, while having two mutated copies causes the genetic disease.

Holandric inheritance Inheritance of genes on Y chromosome. Y-linked genes are only inherited from father to son.

Homologous recombination A type of genetic recombination where nucleotide sequences are exchanged between two similar or identical molecules of nucleic acid. It occurs between paired chromosomes during meiosis and results in genetic variation amongst offspring.

Homozygote/ous An individual with identical alleles at a given locus, or an individual who inherits the same alleles for a particular gene from both parents.

Housekeeping gene These genes express proteins that are essential for basic cellular functions and cell survival. Therefore, they usually have constant levels of expression (constitutive expression).

Human Genome Project (HGP) The Human Genome Project was an international project that mapped and sequenced the entire human genome. Completed in April 2003, data from the project are freely available to researchers and others interested in genetics and human health.

Hybridization The annealing of a single-stranded DNA or RNA molecule to a complementary DNA or RNA sequence.

Idiogram A diagrammatic or schematic version of the karyotype or chromosome complement.

in/del Types of genetic variant; resulting from a small insertion or deletion of nucleotides.

Insulator A DNA element that can act as a barrier or block between a promoter and an enhancer region of a gene.

Intergenic Located between genes on the DNA molecule/chromosome.

Interphase A cell spends most of its time in the cell cycle at the interphase stage, and during this time it grows, replicates its chromosomes, and prepares for cell division.

Intron A portion of a gene that does not code for amino acids. Most human gene sequences are broken up by one or more introns. The parts of the gene sequence that are expressed in the protein are called exons, because they are expressed, while the parts of the gene sequence that are not expressed in the protein are called introns, because they come in between the exons.

In utero In the uterus or in the womb.

Inversion A type of chromosomal abnormality or mutation in which part of a chromosome or DNA sequence is cut and re-joined in a reversed orientation.

In vitro The literal meaning is *in glass* but it also means an experiment or process that takes place in laboratory conditions, e.g. in a test tube or tissue culture dish.

Isochromosome The chromosomal arms of an isochromosome are identical. This is an unbalanced structural chromosome abnormality caused by duplication of one of the chromosome arms.

Isoform One of two or more functionally similar proteins. Can result from alternative splicing.

Karyotype A karyotype is an individual's collection of chromosomes. The term is also commonly used to refer to a laboratory technique that produces an image of an individual's chromosomes. The karyotype is used to look for abnormal numbers or structures of chromosomes.

Liquid biopsy The analysis of cell-free nucleic acid or cells derived from solid tumours. The tumour-derived material is isolated from blood and other bodily fluids, including cerebrospinal fluid and urine.

Matrilineal inheritance Refers to inheritance from the mother or relationships through the female line.

Meiosis Meiosis is a type of cell division that results in the formation of egg and sperm cells. In sexually reproducing organisms, body cells are diploid, meaning they contain two sets of chromosomes (one set from each parent). To maintain this state, the egg and sperm that unite during fertilization must be haploid, meaning they each contain a single set of chromosomes. During meiosis, diploid cells undergo DNA replication, followed by two rounds of cell division, producing four haploid sex cells.

Messenger RNA (mRNA) A single-stranded RNA molecule that is complementary to one of the DNA strands (the template) of a gene. The mRNA is an RNA version of the gene that leaves the cell nucleus and moves to the cytoplasm where proteins are made. During protein synthesis, an organelle called a ribosome moves along the mRNA, reads its base sequence, and uses the genetic code to translate each three-base triplet, or codon, into its corresponding amino acid.

Metacentric (chromosome) Chromosomes with a centromere near the centre, so the p and q arms are of a similar length.

Metaphase Metaphase is a stage during the process of cell division (mitosis or meiosis). Usually, individual chromosomes cannot be observed in the cell nucleus. However, during metaphase of mitosis or meiosis the chromosomes condense and become distinguishable as they align in the centre of the dividing cell. Metaphase chromosomes are analysed during traditional karyotyping procedures that are used to look for chromosomal abnormalities.

Methylation Addition of methyl groups (methylation) is a chemical modification of the DNA molecule. Methylation can change the activity of a

DNA segment without changing the sequence. DNA methylation of a promoter in a gene sequence usually represses gene transcription.

Microarray Probes of nucleic acid sequences (e.g. DNA sequences from across the entire human genome) arranged in a grid pattern for genetic analysis (e.g. hybridization studies).

Mitochondrial inheritance Inheritance of a trait encoded in the mitochondrial genome.

Mitosis Mitosis is a type of cell division. Chromosomes are replicated and two identical nuclei are produced, in preparation for the equal division of the cell nuclei and other cell contents into two daughter cells.

Mixoploid An organism or tissue with different genomes in different cells.

Mobile elements Segments of nucleic acid that can move around within a genome or be transferred from one species to another. These genetic elements are found in all organisms.

Monogenic trait A phenotype or trait that is genetically determined and caused by a variant in one gene. Sometimes referred to as a Mendelian trait, because they follow the laws of heredity described by Gregor Mendel in the nineteenth century.

Monosomy A form of aneuploidy with presence of only one chromosome from a pair.

Multifactorial inheritance Many complex traits are controlled by many genes with additive effects and also influenced by the environment. Multifactorial diseases require the interaction of environmental and additive genetic factors to become manifest.

Multigene family Genes with sequence and functional homology. Genes are derived from a common ancestor through duplication and sequence divergence in evolutionary history.

Mutation hotspot A region of DNA that exhibits an unusually high mutation rate.

Narrow therapeutic index A narrow range between the minimum toxic concentration and the minimum effective concentration of a drug.

Next Generation Sequencing (NGS) High-throughput DNA sequencing methods that are used to determine nucleotide sequence. Many individual methods and laboratory platforms exist for NGS. DNA sequences are analysed in parallel, therefore NGS is sometimes referred to as massively parallel sequencing.

Non-coding (nc) RNA An RNA molecule that is not translated into a protein.

Non-disjunction Homologous chromosomes do not separate during cell division and pass into the same daughter cell. It can result in numerical chromosomal abnormalities, e.g. trisomy.

Non-Invasive Prenatal Diagnosis/Testing (NIPD/NIPT) The prenatal diagnosis of genetic conditions, by analysing circulating fetal DNA in a blood sample taken from the mother.

Nucleotide A nucleotide is the basic building block of nucleic acids. RNA and DNA are polymers made of long chains of nucleotides. A nucleotide consists of a sugar molecule (either ribose in RNA or deoxyribose in DNA) attached to a phosphate group and a nitrogen-containing base. The bases used in DNA are adenine (A), cytosine (C), guanine (G), and thymine (T). In RNA, the base uracil (U) takes the place of thymine.

Okazaki fragments Short lengths of DNA produced during DNA replication on the lagging strand. An enzyme called a DNA ligase joins them to produce a continuous polynucleotide strand.

Oncogene A cancer gene. Genes usually become oncogenes by a mutation that gives them a new or increased function, e.g. *ABL* gene, *ERBB2* gene, *RAS* genes, *MYC* genes. Textbooks often refer to an unmutated version of an oncogene as a proto-oncogene.

Online Mendelian Inheritance in Man (OMIM) An online catalogue describing human genes and genetic disorders. See www.omim.org

Origin of Replication DNA sequence in the genome at which replication is initiated during its synthesis.

Orthologue Genes that are found in different species that evolved from a common ancestral gene. Conserved gene sequence between species.

Paralogue Close resemblance of genes from multigene family. Conserved gene sequence within a species.

Pedigree diagram A diagram to represent family history. Symbols and conventions are used to illustrate phenotypes (and genotypes) for an individual and their relatives over several (usually three or four) generations.

Penetrance The proportion of individuals carrying a particular genetic variant or genotype that also have the associated phenotype. Non-penetrance refers to a clinically unaffected individual who carries the associated mutant genotype.

Pharmacodynamics The study of the effects of drugs and their mechanisms of action.

Pharmacogenetics and pharmacogenomics The study of variability in drug response (both their clinical benefit and adverse effects) due to individual genetic and genome-wide factors.

Pharmacokinetics The study of drug absorption, distribution, metabolism, and excretion.

Pleiotropy A single gene influences two or more independent effects.

Polygenic A polygenic trait is one whose phenotype is influenced by many genes at different loci; each allele exerting a small additive effect. Traits that display a continuous distribution, such as height or skin colour, are polygenic. The inheritance of polygenic traits does not show the phenotypic ratios characteristic of Mendelian inheritance, though each of the genes contributing to the trait is inherited as described by Gregor Mendel. Many polygenic traits are also influenced by the environment and are called multifactorial.

Polygenic risk score A metric that summarizes genome-wide data into a single variable. It is a measure of the known genetic liability for a given phenotype or trait.

Polymerase Chain Reaction (PCR) Polymerase chain reaction (PCR) is a laboratory technique used to amplify DNA sequences. The method involves using short DNA sequences called primers to select the portion of the genome to be amplified. The temperature of the sample is repeatedly raised and lowered to optimize the melting or annealing of DNA, and the activity of the polymerase enzyme to copy the target DNA sequence. The technique can produce a billion copies of the target sequence in less than a couple of hours.

Polymorphism A gene polymorphism describes one of two or more variants of a particular DNA sequence. The term polymorphism is usually used to describe common variants (with a frequency of $\geq$ 1 per cent in a population). The most common type of polymorphism involves variation at a single base pair, called a single nucleotide polymorphism, or SNP (pronounced snip). Scientists are studying how SNPs in the human genome correlate with disease, drug response, and other phenotypes. Polymorphisms can also be much larger in size and involve long stretches of DNA.

Polyploidy A multiple of the haploid chromosome number.

Positional cloning A method used to find the position of a gene associated with a disease on a chromosome by examining the association of markers with the disease, in affected family members (linkage analysis). It requires the identification of partially overlapping DNA segments along the chromosome, near the candidate gene of interest.

Post-translational modification Changes made to protein sequences after synthesis. They include cleavage, glycosylation, phosphorylation, and methylation.

Private mutation A rare gene mutation that may only be observed in a single family or a small population.

Prometaphase A phase of cell division, during which the nuclear envelope breaks down. The duplicated DNA in the parent can then be partitioned into the daughter cells.

Promoter DNA sequence that an RNA polymerase enzyme binds to, to initiate transcription.

Pseudogene A pseudogene is a DNA sequence that resembles a gene but has been mutated over the course of evolution. A pseudogene shares an evolutionary history with a functional gene and can provide insight into their shared ancestry.

Quantitative trait loci (QTL) Loci (positions) in the genome that correlate with a continuous or quantitative trait (a phenotype that varies by degrees) for a given population of individuals.

Reading frame The phase in which nucleotides are read as codons to generate a protein. A single-stranded DNA molecule or mRNA molecule can be read in any of three possible reading frames.

Reference genome sequence The nucleic acid sequence that has been assembled by scientists as a representative example of a species' set of genes. Other genomes are compared with the reference genome sequence to look for genetic variants. It is also referred to as a genome assembly and is updated regularly.

Ribosome A complex cellular particle made of RNA and protein that serves as the site for protein synthesis in the cell. The ribosome reads the sequence of the messenger RNA (mRNA) and, using the genetic code, translates the sequence of RNA bases into a sequence of amino acids.

RNA (Ribonucleic acid) RNA is a single-stranded polynucleotide molecule. An RNA strand has a backbone made of alternating sugar (ribose) and phosphate groups. Attached to each sugar is one of four bases: adenine (A), uracil (U), cytosine (C), or guanine (G). Different types of RNA exist in the cell: e.g. messenger RNA (mRNA), ribosomal RNA (rRNA), and transfer RNA (tRNA), and small nuclear RNAs, which have been found to be involved in regulating gene expression.

Robertsonian translocation A translocation between two acrocentric chromosomes which results in the loss of the genetic material (repetitive DNA sequences) from the short (p) arms.

Semiconservative replication The DNA replication process; one of the original polynucleotide strands remains in each daughter molecule along with only one newly synthesized strand.

Silencer A DNA sequence that a transcription regulatory protein called a repressor can bind to.

Single gene disorder (monogenic disease) Caused by defects in one particular gene, and often have simple and predictable (Mendelian) inheritance patterns.

Single Nucleotide Polymorphism (SNP) Single nucleotide polymorphisms (SNPs, pronounced 'snips') are a type of polymorphism involving variation of a single base pair. Scientists are studying how single nucleotide polymorphisms in the human genome correlate with disease, drug response, and other phenotypes.

Somatic mutation An alteration in DNA that occurs after conception and is not present within the germline. Somatic variants can occur in any of the cells of the body except the germ cells (sperm and egg) and therefore are not passed on to children. Somatic variants can (but do not always) cause cancer or other diseases.

Spliceosome Composed of non-coding RNA and protein, these complex structures excise introns and rejoin exons from pre-mRNA.

Splicing A genetic term describing the production of (diverse) messenger RNA molecules by the differential cutting and joining of molecules from a single precursor RNA.

Statin A commonly prescribed medication used to treat raised cholesterol and to reduce the risk of cardiovascular disease. These are lipid-lowering drugs that inhibit the enzyme HMG CoA reductase. This enzyme plays a central role in the production of cholesterol.

Structural Variant (SV) A type of genetic variant that results from chromosome rearrangements, for example a translocation.

Submetacentric chromosome A chromosome with its centromere located with one chromosome arm shorter than the other.

Superfamily (Gene superfamily) A group of genes (or proteins) with a common ancestry. Their proteins have homologous structural and functional domains.

Tandem repeat A type of DNA variant that can be highly polymorphic (variable between individuals). These are short sequences of DNA that are repeated.

Template strand The double helix of coding DNA consists of a coding strand and a template strand. The template strand is transcribed by RNA Polymerase, which progresses along the template in a 3' to 5' orientation. The template strand of DNA is sometimes referred to as the antisense or non-coding strand.

Termination of Pregnancy (TOP) Medical or surgical termination of pregnancy is legal under particular conditions in many developed countries, including the UK. In the UK's Abortion Act (from 1967), one cause for TOP is *a substantial risk that if a child were born it would suffer from such physical or mental abnormalities as to be seriously handicapped.*

Threshold of Liability The point at which an individual accumulates a liability (which can be monogenic or polygenic and environmental) that means they will be affected by a particular phenotype or disorder.

Thymine A nitrogen-containing pyrimidine base found in DNA.

Topoisomerases Enzymes that have a role in replication and transcription for overwinding and underwinding DNA.

Transcription The production of messenger RNA (mRNA) from a DNA template.

Transcription factors Any protein that initiates or regulates transcription in eukaryotic cells. Transcription factors bind to a variety of regulatory elements for the expression of coding DNA.

Transcriptomics The study of the complete set of RNA transcripts that are produced by the genome, or within a cell or tissue.

Translation The synthesis of a protein sequence from a messenger RNA (mRNA) sequence.

Translocation Translocation is a type of chromosomal abnormality or mutation in which a chromosome breaks and a portion of it reattaches to a different chromosome.

Transposon A DNA sequence that can change position within a genome (sometimes referred to as *jumping genes*).

Trans-regulation The regulation of a gene expression by another (protein or RNA coding) gene. The gene that encodes the regulatory protein or RNA may lie on any chromosome; not necessarily close to the target gene.

Trastuzumab A breast cancer treatment that interferes with a receptor protein (HER-2) over-expressed because of an oncogene (*ERBB2*) mutation. Trastuzumab is a monoclonal antibody treatment used for patients with tumours that express high levels of HER-2 because of the underlying 'driver' oncogene mutation.

Trio analysis Analysis of DNA from both parents and their child to identify genetic variants associated with a phenotype or trait.

Trisomy A numerical chromosome abnormality, with three copies of a chromosome in a cell.

Trisomy 21 A numerical chromosome abnormality, with three copies of chromosome 21 in a cell or karyotype. It is synonymous with the term Down syndrome when used as a title.

Tumour Suppressor Gene (TSG) Often genes that normally prevent or put checks on cell division (control the cell cycle) or genes involved in apoptosis; TSGs are lost or inactivated in cancers. Examples include *P53* & *RB1*.

Uracil A nitrogen-containing pyrimidine base found in RNA.

Variants of Unknown Significance (VUS) A variation in a genetic sequence for which the association with disease risk is unclear. Also called unclassified variant, and variant of uncertain significance.

Warfarin Warfarin is an oral anticoagulant (a drug taken by mouth that stops blood from clotting). It is used to reduce the risk of blood clots, heart attacks, and strokes. Warfarin inhibits the vitamin-K dependent synthesis of blood-clotting factors.

Whole Exome Sequencing (WES) A laboratory process that is used to determine the nucleotide sequence primarily of the exonic (or protein-coding) regions of an individual's genome and related sequences, representing just over 1 per cent of the complete DNA sequence.

Whole Genome Sequencing (WGS) A laboratory process that is used to determine nearly all of the approximately 3 billion nucleotides of an individual's complete DNA sequence, including the non-coding sequence.

X chromosome inactivation (XCI) Male cells have one copy of the X chromosome while female cells have two copies. To prevent female cells from having twice as many gene products from the X chromosomes as males, one copy of the X chromosome in each female cell is inactivated. In placental mammals, the choice of which X chromosome is inactivated is random. XCI is referred to as Lyonization after the geneticist who first described it, Mary Lyon.

X-ray (crystallography) diffraction A technique to determine the molecular structure of a crystal. A beam of X-rays is diffracted. Two-dimensional images of the diffraction pattern can be interpreted as three-dimensional models of crystal structure.

BIBLIOGRAPHY

Chapter 1

Alberts, B., Wilson, J. H., Hunt, T. (2008). *Molecular Biology of the Cell* (5th edn). New York: Garland Science.

Bennett, R. L., French, K. S., Resta, R. G., Doyle, D. L. (2008). Standardized human pedigree nomenclature: update and assessment of the recommendations of the National Society of Genetic Counselors. *Journal of Genetic Counseling*, 17(5), 424–33.

Castel, S. E., Cervera, A., Mohammadi, P., Aguet, F., Reverter, F., *et al.* (2018). Modified penetrance of coding variants by cis-regulatory variation contributes to disease risk. *Nature Genetics*, 50(9), 1327–34.

Franklin, R. E., Gosling, R. G. (1953). Molecular configuration in sodium thymonucleate. *Nature*, 171(4356), 740–1.

Genomes Project Consortium., Abecasis, G. R., Altshuler, D., Auton, A., Brooks, L. D., Durbin, *et al.* (2010). A map of human genome variation from population-scale sequencing. *Nature*, 467(7319), 1061–73.

Hamid, R., Patterson, J., Brandt, S. J. (2008). Genomic structure, alternative splicing and expression of TG-interacting factor, in human myeloid leukemia blasts and cell lines. *Biochimica et Biophysica Acta*, 1779(5), 347–55.

Lander, E. S. (2011). Initial impact of the sequencing of the human genome. *Nature*, 470(7333), 187–97.

Marouli, E., Graff, M., Medina-Gomez, C., Lo, K. S., Wood, A. R., *et al.* (2017). Rare and low-frequency coding variants alter human adult height. *Nature*, 542(7640), 186–90.

Penso-Dolfin, L., Moxon, S., Haerty, W., Di Palma, F. (2018). The evolutionary dynamics of microRNAs in domestic mammals. *Scientific Reports*, 8, Article number: 17050.

Prioleau, M. N., MacAlpine, D. M. (2016). DNA replication origins – where do we begin? *Genes and Development*, 30(15), 1683–97.

Reyes, A., Huber, W. (2018). Alternative start and termination sites of transcription drive most transcript isoform differences across human tissues. *Nucleic acids research*, 46(2), 582–92.

Stark, Z., Dolman, L., Manolio, T. A., Ozenberger, B., Hill, S. L., *et al.* (2019). Integrating Genomics into Healthcare: A Global Responsibility *American Journal of Human Genetics*, 104(1), 13–20.

Turnpenny, P. D., Ellard, S. (2017). *Emery's Elements of Medical Genetics*. Amsterdam: Elsevier.

Watson, J. D., Crick, F. H. (1953). Molecular structure of nucleic acids; a structure for deoxyribose nucleic acid. *Nature*, 171(4356), 737–8.

Wood, A. R., Esko, T., Yang, J., Vedantam, S., Pers, T. H., *et al.* (2014). Defining the role of common variation in the genomic and biological architecture of adult human height. *Nature Genetics*, 46(11), 1173–86.

Xue, Y., Wang, Q., Long, Q., Ng, B. L., Swerdlow, *et al.* (2009). Human Y chromosome base-substitution mutation rate measured by direct sequencing in a deep-rooting pedigree. *Current Biology*, 19(17), 1453–7.

Chapter 2

Acuna-Hidalgo, R., Veltman, J. A., Hoischen, A. (2016). New insights into the generation and role of de novo mutations in health and disease. *Genome Biology*, 17(1), Article No. 241.

Alberts, B., Wilson, J. H., Hunt, T. (2008). *Molecular Biology of the Cell* (5th edn). New York: Garland Science.

Bennett, R. L., French, K. S., Resta, R. G., Doyle, D. L. *et al.* (2008). Standardized human pedigree nomenclature: update and assessment of the recommendations of the National Society of Genetic Counselors. *Journal of Genetic Counseling*, 17(5), 424–33.

Buniello, A., MacArthur, J. A. L., Cerezo, M., Harris, L. W., Hayhurst, J. *et al.* (2019). The NHGRI-EBI GWAS Catalog of published genome-wide association studies, targeted arrays and summary statistics 2019. *Nucleic Acids Research*, 47(D1), D1005–D1012.

den Dunnen, J. T., Dalgleish, R., Maglott, D. R., Hart, R. K., Greenblatt, M. S. *et al.* (2016). HGVS Recommendations for the Description of Sequence Variants: 2016 Update. *Human Mutation*, 37(6), 564–9.

Feder, J. N., Gnirke, A., Thomas, W., Tsuchihashi, Z., Ruddy, D. A. *et al.* (1996). A novel MHC class I-like gene is mutated in patients with hereditary haemochromatosis. *Nature Genetics*, 13(4), 399–408.

Genomes Project, C., Auton, A., Brooks, L. D., Durbin, R. M., Garrison, E. P. *et al.* (2015). A global reference for human genetic variation. *Nature*, 526(7571), 68–74. doi:10.1038/nature15393

Helleday, T., Eshtad, S., Nik-Zainal, S. (2014). Mechanisms underlying mutational signatures in human cancers. *Nature Reviews Genetics*, 15(9), 585–98.

Lander, E. S. (2011). Initial impact of the sequencing of the human genome. *Nature*, 470(7333), 187–97.

Online Mendelian Inheritance in Man, OMIM®. (n.d.). McKusick–Nathans Institute of Genetic Medicine, Johns Hopkins University (Baltimore, MD), (January 2020): https://omim.org/

Purandare, S. M., Patel, P. I. (1997). Recombination hot spots and human disease. *Genome Research*, 7(8), 773–86.

Timpson, N. J., Greenwood, C. M. T., Soranzo, N., Lawson, D. J., Richards, J. B. (2018). Genetic architecture: the shape of the genetic contribution to human traits and disease. *Nature Reviews Genetics*, 19(2), 110–24.

Turnpenny, P. D., Ellard, S. (2017). *Emery's Elements of Medical Genetics*. Amsterdam: Elsevier.

Xue, Y., Wang, Q., Long, Q., Ng, B. L., Swerdlow, H., *et al.* (2009). Human Y chromosome base-substitution mutation rate measured by direct sequencing in a deep-rooting pedigree. *Current Biology*, 19(17), 1453–7.

Yates, B., Braschi, B., Gray, K. A., Seal, R. L., Tweedie, S., *et al.* (2017). Genenames.org: the HGNC and VGNC resources in 2017. *Nucleic Acids Research*, 45(D1), D619–D625.

Chapter 3

Ashley, E. A. (2016). Towards precision medicine. *Nature Reviews Genetics*, 17(9), 507–22.

Bentley, D. R., Balasubramanian, S., Swerdlow, H. P., Smith, G. P., Milton, J., *et al.* (2008). Accurate whole human genome sequencing using reversible terminator chemistry. *Nature*, 456(7218), 53–9.

Evans, J. P., Powell, B. C., Berg, J. S. (2017). Finding the Rare Pathogenic Variants in a Human Genome. *Journal of the American Medical Association*, 317(18), 1904–5.

Hadfield, J. (2014). The application of genomic technologies to cancer and companion diagnostics. PhD dissertation, University of East Anglia. Retrieved from: https://ueaeprints.uea.ac.uk/53447

Hayden, E. C. (2014). Technology: The $1,000 genome. *Nature*, 507(7492), 294–5.

Houge, G., Haesen, D., Vissers, L. E., Mehta, S., Parker, M. J., *et al.* (2015). B56delta-related protein phosphatase 2A dysfunction identified in patients with intellectual disability. *Journal of Clinical Investigation*, 125(8), 3051–62.

Lam, H. Y., Clark, M. J., Chen, R., Chen, R., Natsoulis, G., *et al.* (2012). Performance comparison of whole-genome sequencing platforms. *Nature Biotechnology*, 30(1), 78–82.

Mullis, K., Faloona, F., Scharf, S., Saiki, R., Horn, G., *et al.* (1986). Specific enzymatic amplification of DNA in vitro: the polymerase chain reaction. *Cold Spring Harbour Symposia on Quantitative Biology*, 51 Pt 1, 263–73.

Nuffield Council on Bioethics Non-invasive prenatal testing. Retrieved January 2020 from: https://nuffieldbioethics.org/publications/non-invasive-prenatal-testing

Online Mendelian Inheritance in Man, OMIM®. (n.d.). McKusick–Nathans Institute of Genetic Medicine, Johns Hopkins University, Baltimore, MD. Retrieved January 2020 from: https://omim.org

Richards, S., Aziz, N., Bale, S., Bick, D., Das, S., *et al.* Committee, ACMG Laboratory Quality Assurance Committee (2015). Standards and guidelines for the interpretation of sequence variants: a joint consensus recommendation of the American College of Medical Genetics and Genomics and the Association for Molecular Pathology. *Genetics in Medicine*, 17(5), 405–24.

Chapter 4

Abascal, F., Juan, D., Jungreis, I., Martinez, L., Rigau, M., *et al.* (2018). Loose ends: almost one in five human genes still have unresolved coding status. *Nucleic Acids Research*, 46(14), 7070–84.

Acuna-Hidalgo, R., Veltman, J. A., Hoischen, A. (2016). New insights into the generation and role of de novo mutations in health and disease. *Genome Biology*, 17(1), 241.

Bennett, R. L., French, K. S., Resta, R. G., Doyle, D. L. (2008). Standardized human pedigree nomenclature: update and assessment of the recommendations of the National Society of Genetic Counselors. *Journal of Genetic Counseling*, 17(5), 424–33.

FDNA. (2019). Redefining phenotyping for clinical advancements and variant prioritization. Retrieved January 2020 from: https://www.fdna.com/fdnainsights/?_ga=2.89802514.888731833.1560687632-100998475.1560687632

Gravholt, C. H., Chang, S., Wallentin, M., Fedder, J., Moore, P., *et al.* (2018). Klinefelter Syndrome: integrating genetics, neuropsychology, and endocrinology. *Endocrine Reviews*, 39(4), 389–423.

Health Education England's Genomics Education Programme (GEP). (n.d.). Retrieved January 2020 from: https://www.genomicseducation.hee.nhs.uk/using-our-content

Houge, G., Haesen, D., Vissers, L. E., Mehta, S., Parker, M. J., *et al.* (2015). B56delta-related protein phosphatase 2A dysfunction identified in patients with intellectual disability. *Journal of Clinical Investigation*, 125(8), 3051–62.

Meyer, R. E., Liu, G., Gilboa, S. M., Ethen, M. K., Aylsworth, A. S., *et al.* National Birth Defects Prevention (2016). Survival of children with trisomy 13 and trisomy 18: A multi-state population-based study. *American Journal of Medical Genetics*, 170A(4), 825–37.

Mutai, H., Watabe, T., Kosaki, K., Ogawa, K., Matsunaga, T. (2017). Mitochondrial mutations in maternally inherited hearing loss. *BMC Medical Genetics*, 18(1), 32. doi:10.1186/s12881-017-0389-4

Online Mendelian Inheritance in Man, OMIM®. (n.d.). McKusick–Nathans Institute of Genetic Medicine, Johns Hopkins University, Baltimore, MD. Retrieved January 2020 from: https://omim.org

Purandare, S. M., Patel, P. I. (1997). Recombination hot spots and human disease. *Genome Research*, 7(8), 773–86.

Richards, S., Aziz, N., Bale, S., Bick, D., Das, S., *et al.* Committee, ACMG Laboratory Quality Assurance Committee (2015). Standards and guidelines for the interpretation of sequence variants: a joint consensus recommendation of the American College of Medical Genetics and Genomics and the Association for Molecular Pathology. *Genetics in Medicine*, 17(5), 405–24.

Robinson, A., Linden, M. G. (1993). *Clinical Genetics Handbook* (2nd edn). Boston, MA and Oxford: Blackwell Scientific Publications.

Shankar, R. K., Backeljauw, P. F. (2018). Current best practice in the management of Turner syndrome. *Therapeutic Advances in Endocrinology and Metabolism*, 9(1), 33–40.

Tanaka, A. J., Sauer, M. V., Egli, D., Kort, D. H. (2013). Harnessing the stem cell potential: the path to prevent mitochondrial disease. *Nature Medicine*, 19(12), 1578–9.

Timpson, N. J., Greenwood, C. M. T., Soranzo, N., Lawson, D. J., Richards, J. B. (2018). Genetic architecture: the shape of the genetic contribution to human traits and disease. *Nature Reviews Genetics*, 19(2), 110–24.

Turnbull, C., Scott, R. H., Thomas, E., Jones, L., Murugaesu, N., *et al.* (2018). The 100 000 Genomes Project: bringing whole genome sequencing to the NHS. *BMJ*, 361, k1687.

Turnpenny, P. D., Ellard, S. (2017). *Emery's Elements of Medical Genetics*. Amsterdam: Elsevier.

Vega, A. I., Medrano, C., Navarrete, R., Desviat, L. R., Merinero, B., *et al.* (2016). Molecular diagnosis of glycogen storage disease and disorders with overlapping clinical symptoms by massive parallel sequencing. *Genetics in Medicine*, 18(10), 1037–43.

Warsy, A. S., Al-Jaser, M. H., Albdass, A., Al-Daihan, S., Alanazi, M. (2014). Is consanguinity prevalence decreasing in Saudis? A study in two generations. *African Health Sciences*, 14(2), 314–21.

Wright, C. F., FitzPatrick, D. R., Firth, H. V. (2018). Paediatric genomics: diagnosing rare disease in children. *Nature Reviews Genetics*, 19(5), 253–68.

Xue, Y., Wang, Q., Long, Q., Ng, B. L., Swerdlow, H., *et al.* (2009). Human Y chromosome base-substitution mutation rate measured by direct sequencing in a deep-rooting pedigree. *Current Biology*, 19(17), 1453–7.

Yang, Y., Muzny, D. M., Reid, J. G., Bainbridge, M. N., Willis, A., *et al.* (2013). Clinical whole-exome sequencing for the diagnosis of mendelian disorders. *New England Journal of Medicine*, 369(16), 1502–11.

Chapter 5

Aretz, S., Vasen, H. F., Olschwang, S. (2015). Clinical Utility Gene Card for: Familial adenomatous polyposis (FAP) and attenuated FAP (AFAP) – update 2014. *European Journal of Human Genetics*, 23(6).

Berkowitz, C. L., Mosconi, L., Scheyer, O., Rahman, A., Hristov, H., *et al.* (2018). Precision medicine for Alzheimer's disease prevention. *Healthcare (Basel)*, 6(3), 82.

Bardou-Jacquet, E., Laine, F., Deugnier, Y. (2015). Reply to: 'Reduced mortality due to phlebotomy in moderately iron-loaded HFE Haemochromatosis? The need for clinical trials'. *Journal of Hepatology*, 63(1), 283–4.

Bardou-Jacquet, E., Morcet, J., Manet, G., Lainé, F., Perrin, M. *et al.* (2015). Decreased cardiovascular and extrahepatic cancer-related mortality in treated patients with mild HFE hemochromatosis. *Journal of Hepatology*, 62(3), 682–9.

Claussnitzer, M., Cho, J. H., Collins, R., Cox, N. J., Dermitzakis, E. T., *et al.* (2020). A brief history of human disease genetics. *Nature*, 577, 179–89.

Deugnier, Y., Morcet, J., Laine, F., Hamdi-Roze, H., Bollard, A..S., *et al.* (2019). Reduced phenotypic expression in genetic hemochromatosis with time: role of exposure to nongenetic modifiers. *Journal of Hepatology*, 70(1),118–25.

Dudley, J. T. Karczewski K. J. (2014). *Exploring Personal Genomics*. Oxford: Oxford University Press.

Evans, J. P., Powell, B. C., Berg, J. S. (2017). Finding the Rare Pathogenic Variants in a Human Genome. *Journal of the American Medical Association*, 317(18), 1904–5.

Findlay, G. M., Daza, R. M., Martin, B., Zhang, M. D., Leith, A. P., *et al.* (2018). Accurate classification of BRCA1 variants with saturation genome editing. *Nature*, 562(7726), 217–22.

Gottesman, I. I. Erlenmeyer-Kimling, L. (2001). Family and twin strategies as a head start in defining prodromes and endophenotypes for hypothetical early-interventions in schizophrenia. *Schizophrenia Research*, 51(1), 93–102.

Grosse, S. D., Gurrin, L. C., Bertalli, N. A., Allen, K. J. (2018) Clinical penetrance in hereditary hemochromatosis: estimates of the cumulative incidence of severe liver disease among HFE C282Y homozygotes. *Genetics in Medicine*, 20(4), 383–9.

Khera, A. V., Kathiresan, S. (2017). Genetics of coronary artery disease: discovery, biology and clinical translation. *Nature Reviews Genetics*, 18(6), 331–44.

Maeder, M. L. M., Stefanidakis, C. J., Wilson, R., Baral, L. A., Barrera, G. S., *et al.* (2019). Development of a gene-editing approach to restore vision loss in Leber congenital amaurosis type 10. *Nature Medicine*, 25(2), 229–33

Marouli, E., Graff, M., Medina-Gomez, C., *et al.* (2017). Rare and low-frequency coding variants alter human adult height. *Nature*, 542(7640), 186–90.

Ong, S. Y., Dolling, L., Dixon, J. L., Nicoll, A. J., Gurrinet, L.C., *et al.* (2015). Should HFE p.C282Y homozygotes with moderately elevated serum ferritin be treated? A randomised controlled trial comparing iron reduction with sham treatment (Mi-iron). *The BMJ Open*, 5(8), e008938.

Pilling, L. C., Tamosauskaite, J., Jones, G., Wood, A. R., Jones, L., *et al.* (2019). Common conditions associated with hereditary haemochromatosis genetic variants: cohort study in UK Biobank. *The BMJ (Clinical Research Edn)* 364, k5222.

Plomin, R. (2018). *Blueprint: How DNA Makes Us Who We Are*. Harmondsworth: Allen Lane (Penguin).

Stuhrmann, M., Gabriel, H., Keeney, S. (2010). Clinical utility gene card for: Haemochromatosis [HFE]. *European Journal of Human Genetics*, 2010, 18(9).

Willemsen, G., Ward, K. J., Bell, C. G., Christensen, K., Bowden, J., *et al.* (2015). The Concordance and Heritability of Type 2 Diabetes in 34,166 Twin Pairs From International Twin Registers: The Discordant Twin (DISCOTWIN) Consortium. *Twin Research and Human Genetics*, 18(6), 762–71.

Wood, A. R., Esko, T., Yang, J., Vedantam, S., Pers, T. H., *et al.* (2014). Defining the role of common variation in the genomic and biological architecture of adult human height. *Nature Genetics*, 46(11), 1173–86.

Chapter 6

Aklillu, E., Persson, I., Bertilsson, L., Johansson, I., Rodrigues, F., *et al.* (1996). Frequent distribution of ultrarapid metabolizers of debrisoquine in an Ethiopian population carrying duplicated and multiduplicated functional CYP2D6 alleles. *Journal of Pharmacology and Experimental Therapeutics*, 278(1), 441–6.

Dudley, J. T., Karczewski, K. J. (2013). *Exploring Personal Genomics*. Oxford: Oxford University Press.

Feiler, T., Gaitskell, K., Maughan, T., Hordern, J. (2017). Personalised medicine: the promise, the hype and the pitfalls. *The New Bioethics*, 23(1), 1–12.

Hetherington, S., Hughes, A. R., Mosteller, M., Shortino, D., Baker, K. L., *et al.* (2002). Genetic variations in HLA-B region and hypersensitivity reactions to abacavir. *Lancet*, 359(9312), 1121–2.

Jennings, B. A., Shakespeare, T., Loke, Y. K. (2015). Scanning the human genome and the horizon: the potential and pitfalls of pharmacogenetics and stratified medicine. *British Journal of General Practice*, 65(635), 284–5.

Kelly, L. E., Rieder, M., van den Anker, J., Malkin, B., Ross, C., *et al.* (2012). More codeine fatalities after tonsillectomy in North American children. *Pediatrics*, 129(5), e1343–1347.

Manuchair, E. (2008). *Desk Reference of Clinical Pharmacology*. Abingdon: CRC Press, Taylor & Francis Group.

Meulendijks, D., Henricks, L. M., Sonke, G. S., Deenen, M. J., Froehlich, T. K., *et al.* (2015). Clinical relevance of DPYD variants c.1679T>G, c.1236G>A/HapB3, and c.1601G>A as predictors of severe fluoropyrimidine-associated toxicity: a systematic review and meta-analysis of individual patient data. *Lancet Oncology*, 16(16), 1639–50.

Murtaza, M., Dawson, S. J., Tsui, D. W., Gale, D., Forshew, T., *et al.* (2013). Non-invasive analysis of acquired resistance to cancer therapy by sequencing of plasma DNA. *Nature*, 497(7447), 108–12.

Rattanavipapong, W., Koopitakkajorn, T., Praditsitthikorn, N., Mahasirimongkol, S., Teerawattananon, Y. (2013). Economic evaluation of HLA-B*15:02 screening for carbamazepine-induced severe adverse drug reactions in Thailand. *Epilepsia*, 54(9), 1628–38.

Relling, M. V., Evans, W. E. (2015). Pharmacogenomics in the clinic. *Nature*, 526(7573), 343–50.

Schully, S. D., Benedicto, C. B., Khoury, M. J. (2012). How can we stimulate translational research in cancer genomics beyond bench to bedside? *Genetics in Medicine*, 14(1), 169–70.

Soreide, K. (2009). Receiver-operating characteristic curve analysis in diagnostic, prognostic and predictive biomarker research. *Journal of Clinical Pathology*, 62(1), 1–5.

Stergiopoulos, K., Brown, D. L. (2014). Genotype-guided vs clinical dosing of warfarin and its analogues: meta-analysis of randomized clinical trials. *JAMA Internal Medicine*, 174(8), 1330–8.

Thorn, C. F., Marsh, S., Carrillo, M. W., McLeod, H. L., Klein, T. E., *et al.* (2011). PharmGKB summary: fluoropyrimidine pathways. *Pharmacogenetics and Genomics*, 21(4), 237–42.

Usui, T., Naisbitt, D. J. (2017). Human leukocyte antigen and idiosyncratic adverse drug reactions. *Drug Metabolism and Pharmacokinetics*, 32(1), 21–30.

Whirl-Carrillo, M., McDonagh, E. M., Hebert, J. M., Gong, L., Sangkuhl, K., *et al.* (2012). Pharmacogenomics knowledge for personalized medicine. *Clinical Pharmacology and Therapeutics*, 92(4), 414–17.

INDEX

Note: Figures and Tables are cross referred in the Index.